ONE STOP DOC

Metabolism and Nutrition

One Stop Doc

Titles in the series include:

Cardiovascular System – Jonathan Aron
Editorial Advisor – Jeremy Ward

Cell and Molecular Biology – Desikan Rangarajan and David Shaw
Editorial Advisor – Barbara Moreland

Endocrine and Reproductive Systems – Caroline Jewels and Alexandra Tillett
Editorial Advisor – Stuart Milligan

Gastrointestinal System – Miruna Canagaratnam
Editorial Advisor – Richard Naftalin

Musculoskeletal System – Wayne Lam, Bassel Zebian and Rishi Aggarwal
Editorial Advisor – Alistair Hunter

Nervous System – Elliott Smock
Editorial Advisor – Clive Coen

Renal and Urinary System and Electrolyte Balance – Panos Stamoulos and Spyridon Bakalis
Editorial Advisors – Alistair Hunter and Richard Naftalin

Respiratory System – Jo Dartnell and Michelle Ramsay
Editorial Advisor – John Rees

ONE STOP DOC
Metabolism and Nutrition

Miruna Canagaratnam BSc(Hons)
Fifth year medical student, Guy's, King's and
St Thomas' Medical School, London, UK

David Shaw BSc(Hons)
Fifth year medical student, Guy's, King's and
St Thomas' Medical School, London, UK

Editorial Advisor: Barbara Moreland BSc(Hons) PhD
Senior Lecturer, Division of Biomedical Sciences, Guy's, King's and
St Thomas' School of Biomedical Sciences, London, UK

Editorial Advisor: Richard J. Naftalin MB ChB MSc PhD DSc
Professor of Epithelial Physiology, King's College, London,
Guy's Campus Centre for Vascular Biology and Medicine, London, UK

Series Editor: Elliott Smock BSc(Hons)
Fifth year medical student, Guy's, King's and
St Thomas' Medical School, London, UK

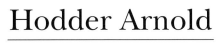

Hodder Arnold

A MEMBER OF THE HODDER HEADLINE GROUP

First published in Great Britain in 2005 by
Hodder Education, a member of the Hodder Headline Group,
338 Euston Road, London NW1 3BH

http://www.hoddereducation.co.uk

Distributed in the United States of America by
Oxford University Press Inc.,
198 Madison Avenue, New York, NY10016
Oxford is a registered trademark of Oxford University Press

Whilst the advice and information in this book are believed to be true and
accurate at the date of going to press, neither the authors nor the publisher
can accept any legal responsibility or liability for any errors or omissions
that may be made. In particular, (but without limiting the generality of the
preceding disclaimer) every effort has been made to check drug dosages;
however it is still possible that errors have been missed. Furthermore,
dosage schedules are constantly being revised and new side-effects
recognized. For these reasons the reader is strongly urged to consult the
drug companies' printed instructions before administering any of the drugs
recommended in this book.

British Library Cataloguing in Publication Data
A catalogue record for this book is available from the British Library

Library of Congress Cataloging-in-Publication Data
A catalog record for this book is available from the Library of Congress

ISBN-10: 0 340 88940 3
ISBN-13: 978 0 340 88940 4

1 2 3 4 5 6 7 8 9 10

Commissioning Editor: Georgina Bentliff
Project Editor: Heather Smith
Production Controller: Jane Lawrence
Cover Design: Amina Dudhia
Illustrations: Cactus Design

Hodder Headline's policy is to use papers that are natural, renewable and recyclable
products and made from wood grown in sustainable forests. The logging and manufacturing processes are
expected to conform to the environmental regulations of the country of origin.

Typeset in 10/12pt Adobe Garamond/Akzidenz GroteskBE by Servis Filmsetting Ltd, Manchester
Printed and bound in Spain

What do you think about this book? Or any other Hodder Arnold title?
Please visit our website at **www.hoddereducation.co.uk**

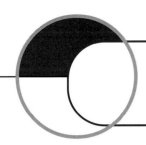

CONTENTS

PREFACE   vi

ABBREVIATIONS   vii

SECTION 1   ENERGY METABOLISM   1

SECTION 2   LIPID AND AMINO ACID METABOLISM   27

SECTION 3   METABOLIC INTEGRATION AND METABOLIC DISORDERS   55

SECTION 4   GENERAL NUTRITION   79

SECTION 5   CLINICAL ASPECTS OF NUTRITION   97

INDEX   113

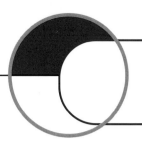

PREFACE

FROM THE SERIES EDITOR, ELLIOTT SMOCK

Are you ready to face your looming exams? If you have done loads of work, then congratulations; we hope this opportunity to practice SAQs, EMQs, MCQs and Problem-based Questions on every part of the core curriculum will help you consolidate what you've learnt and improve your exam technique. If you don't feel ready, don't panic – the One Stop Doc series has all the answers you need to catch up and pass.

There are only a limited number of questions an examiner can throw at a beleaguered student and this text can turn that to your advantage. By getting straight into the heart of the core questions that come up year after year and by giving you the model answers you need this book will arm you with the knowledge to succeed in your exams. Broken down into logical sections, you can learn all the important facts you need to pass without having to wade through tons of different textbooks when you simply don't have the time. All questions presented here are 'core'; those of the highest importance have been highlighted to allow even sharper focus if time for revision is running out. In addition, to allow you to organize your revision efficiently, questions have been grouped by topic, with answers supported by detailed integrated explanations.

On behalf of all the One Stop Doc authors I wish you the very best of luck in your exams and hope these books serve you well!

FROM THE AUTHORS, MIRUNA CANAGARATNAM AND DAVID SHAW

Metabolism and Nutrition can seem a daunting subject when confronted for the first time. This book breaks the subject down into small chunks and aims to put a clinical perspective on the basic science, so that you can understand it better for both the exams and your career.

The book is divided into five sections: Energy metabolism, Lipid and amino acid metabolism, Metabolic integration and metabolic disorders, General nutrition and Clinical aspects of nutrition. Each section is covered through MCQs, EMQs, SAQs and clinical cases where you can apply your basic knowledge.

We would like to extend many heartfelt thanks to Professor Naftalin and Dr Moreland for their unfailing support and hard work in shaping this book. We are eternally grateful for their help and expertise. Thanks again to Elliott for his good advice and excellent mediation skills. Thank you too to Heather Smith for her patience and understanding.

We hope this book helps you, not only to gain a good grasp of Metabolism and Nutrition, but also to enjoy it!

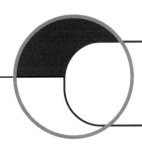

ABBREVIATIONS

ADP	adenosine diphosphate
ALT	alanine aminotransferase
AMP	adenosine monophosphate
apo	apoprotein
AST	aspartate aminotransferase
ATP	adenosine triphosphate
AMP	adenosine monophosphate
BMI	body mass index
BMR	basal metabolic rate
cAMP	cyclic adenosine monophosphate
2,3-BPG	2,3-bisphosphoglycerate
CHD	coronary heart disease
CNS	central nervous system
DHAP	dihydroxyacetone phosphate
DNA	deoxyribonucleic acid
DRV	dietary reference value
EAR	estimated average requirement
FA	fatty acid
FAD	flavine adenine dinucleotide
FADH$_2$	reduced form of flavine adenine dinucleotide
FFA	free fatty acid
FMN	flavine mononucleotide
G6PD	glucose 6-phosphate dehydrogenase
GDP	guanosine diphosphate
GI	gastrointestinal
GP	general practitioner
GSH	reduced glutathione
GS-SG	oxidized glutathione
GTP	guanosine triphosphate
3HBD	3-hydroxybutyrate dehydrogenase
HDL	high density lipoprotein
HIV	human immunodeficiency virus
HMG CoA	3-hydroxy-3-methylglutaryl CoA

IgA	immunoglobulin A
IgE	immunoglobulin E
IDL	intermediate density lipoprotein
KB	ketone body
LCAT	lecithin:cholesterol acyltransferase
LDL	low density lipoprotein
MDH	malate dehydrogenase
NAD	nicotinamide adenine dinucleotide
NAD$^+$	oxidized form of nicotinamide adenine dinucleotide
NADH	reduced form of nicotinamide adenine dinucleotide
NADP	nicotinamide adenine dinucleotide phosphate
NADP$^+$	oxidized form of nicotinamide adenine dinucleotide phosphate
NADPH	reduced form of nicotinamide adenine dinucleotide phosphate
NSAID	non-steroidal anti-inflammatory drug
PEM	protein energy malnutrition
PKU	phenylketonuria
PPi	pyrophosphate
Pi	inorganic phosphate
RBC	red blood cell
RNI	reference nutrient intake
TAG	triacylglycerol
TCA	tricarboxylic acid
THF	tetrahydrofolate
UDP	uridine diphosphate
UTP	uridine triphosphate
UV	ultraviolet
VLDL	very low density lipoprotein

1   ENERGY METABOLISM

- METABOLIC RATE   2
- GLUCOSE METABOLISM   4, 26
- GLYCOLYSIS (i)   6
- GLYCOLYSIS (ii)   8
- REGULATION OF GLYCOLYSIS   10
- GLYCOGEN – STRUCTURE AND SYNTHESIS   12
- DISORDERS OF GLYCOGEN STORAGE   14
- THE CITRIC ACID CYCLE   16
- METABOLIC IMPORTANCE OF CITRIC ACID CYCLE   18
- OXIDATIVE PHOSPHORYLATION   20
- GLUCONEOGENESIS (i)   22
- GLUCONEOGENESIS (ii)   24

ENERGY METABOLISM

1. Which of the following factors affect metabolic rate?

a. Environmental temperature
b. Circulating insulin levels
c. Muscle exertion during or before measurement
d. Recent ingestion of food
e. Age

2. The basal metabolic rate of a man

a. Is never greater than 1000 kcal/day
b. Can be determined 2 hours after his last meal
c. Falls during prolonged starvation
d. Falls immediately after feeding
e. Rises during fever

BMR, basal metabolic rate

EXPLANATION: METABOLIC RATE

Metabolic rate is usually determined by measuring **oxygen consumption**. Therefore it is natural that **muscular exertion** would be a major factor affecting metabolic rate.

Another factor to consider is **environmental temperature**. If it falls below body temperature, heat conserving mechanisms kick in (i.e. **cutaneous vasoconstriction** and **shivering**). This causes the metabolic rate to rise. When environmental temperature increases to a point where it is high enough to raise body temperature, **metabolic enzyme** action accelerates. Therefore **metabolic rate rises with an increase in body temperature**.

Other factors affecting metabolic rate include **emotional state**, **height**, **weight** and circulating levels of hormones such as **adrenaline** and **thyroxine**, but not insulin.

BMR is a measure of the energy requirement for the **maintenance** of metabolic integrity, nerve and muscle tone, circulation and respiration in the human body under controlled conditions of thermal neutrality. The BMR of an average sized man is about **2000 kcal/day**. A normal BMR in an adult male is around 40 kcal/m^2/h. The BMR falls during prolonged starvation due to loss of skeletal muscle bulk. A high fever increases BMR.

In comparison to males BMR is generally **lower** in females and **higher** in children. BMR is measured 12–14 hours after a meal, by direct or indirect calorimetry. Feeding increases BMR because of the necessary energy expenditure that occurs during the assimilation of nutrients into the body (also known as **specific dynamic action**). BMR is also very closely related to **body surface area**, since this is where the majority of heat exchange takes place.

Answers
1. T F T T T
2. F F T F T

3. True or false? Glucose

a. Is the only fuel source for erythrocytes
b. Cannot cross the blood–brain barrier
c. Enters cells through simple diffusion through the cell membrane
d. Is phosphorylated in the liver by glucokinase
e. In high concentrations may directly damage cells

4. The conversion of glucose to pyruvate

a. Produces 31 molecules of ATP per glucose molecule
b. Occurs outside the mitochondria
c. Is reversible
d. Requires the enzyme pyruvate kinase
e. Requires the phosphorylation of glucose

5. Put the steps of glycolysis in the correct order

A. Formation of pyruvate
B. 3-Phosphoglycerate is converted to 2-phosphoglycerate
C. Cleavage of fructose 1,6-bisphosphate
D. Reduction of NAD^+
E. Phosphorylation of glucose
F. Dehydration of 2-phosphoglycerate to phosphoenolpyruvate

ATP, adenosine triphosphate; RBC, red blood cell; NAD^+, oxidized form of nicotinamide adenine dinucleotide; TCA, tricarboxylic acid

EXPLANATION: GLUCOSE METABOLISM

Glucose is the favoured fuel source of **all tissues**. Physiological concentration of glucose in the blood is tightly regulated to stay within the normal range of 3.9–6.7 mmol/L. If blood glucose drops to below 2.7 mmol/L **hypoglycaemia** reduces the energy available to the vital organs, which can lead to **coma** and **death**. The main advantages of glucose as a metabolic fuel are that it is **water soluble**, it can cross the **blood–brain barrier** and it can be oxidized **anaerobically**. However, it also yields a relatively small amount of ATP compared to other fuels, and is **osmotically active**, thus it can **damage** cells. Glucose is the only fuel for RBCs, which have no mitochondria.

Glucose transport across membranes occurs via a transporter protein, i.e. GLUT transporters. These transmembrane proteins bind glucose on one face of the membrane, then undergo conformational change to translocate glucose across the membrane. The different types of GLUT transporter are outlined in the table below:

Transporter	Location
GLUT 1	Erythrocyte, kidney
GLUT 2	Intestinal epithelial cells, liver and kidney
GLUT 3	Neurons, i.e. brain
GLUT 4	Adipose tissue, muscle
GLUT 5	Intestinal epithelial cells and kidney

Co-transporter	Location
SGLT 1	Small intestine
SGLT 2	Renal tubules

Glycolysis is the process by which **glucose** is converted to **pyruvate** to enter the TCA cycle. **Two ATP** molecules are produced per molecule of glucose that enters the pathway. There are three irreversible steps in glycolysis, catalysed by the following enzymes: **hexokinase/glucokinase**, **phosphofructokinase** and **pyruvate kinase**.

Glycolysis that occurs in the presence of **oxygen** produces **pyruvate** which can then enter the TCA cycle to produce CO_2. It is performed by all tissues. Glycolysis can occur in the **absence** of **oxygen** to produce **lactate** (anaerobic). Anaerobic glycolysis allows cells that lack mitochondria to produce ATP, for example RBCs. Remember, pyruvate/lactate formation takes place in the cytosol **not** the mitochondria.

See page 26 for a summary diagram of glucose metabolism **(5)**.

Answers
3. T F F T T
4. F T T T T
5. 1 – E, 2 – C, 3 – D, 4 – B, 5 – F, 6 – A (see diagram page 26)

6. True or false? Glycolysis

    a. Always requires oxygen
    b. Can only occur in erythrocytes
    c. Requires more energy than it produces
    d. Is inhibited by insulin
    e. Occurs inside the mitochondria

7. An inherited deficiency of pyruvate kinase

    a. Is the most common glycolytic enzyme deficiency
    b. Causes destruction of red blood cells
    c. Causes a rise in lactate formation
    d. Is associated with a rise in ADP:ATP ratio
    e. Affects the metabolism of all tissues

8. True or false? Glucokinase

    a. Is found in the liver and beta cells of the pancreas
    b. Has a low K_m (high affinity) for glucose
    c. Is inhibited by glucose 6-phosphate
    d. Is specific to glucose as a substrate
    e. Levels are increased by insulin

ADP, adenosine diphosphate; ATP, adenosine triphosphate

EXPLANATION: GLYCOLYSIS (i)

Pyruvate kinase catalyses the **formation** of **pyruvate** from phosphoenolpyruvate in the glycolysis pathway, with the production of **two molecules of ATP**. People with a relatively common inherited deficiency of pyruvate kinase demonstrate haemolytic anaemia due to the inadequate production of ATP by glycolysis to meet the erythrocytes' energy needs. Since the cell has no other method of producing ATP, it is unable to maintain the structural integrity of its cell membrane. This leads to changes in the shape of the red blood cell and hence its destruction by phagocytosis.

Glucokinase catalyses the first reaction of **glycolysis** in the liver – the phosphorylation of glucose. Glucokinase differs from hexokinase, the enzyme used in all other tissues, in that it requires a higher concentration of glucose to become half-saturated (**high K_m**). It only functions when glucose concentration in the liver is very high, in other words directly after a carbohydrate-rich meal. This allows the liver to **remove glucose** from the **portal blood effectively** preventing hyperglycaemia.

The main differences between glucokinase and hexokinase are listed below:

Glucokinase	Hexokinase
Liver and beta cells in pancreas	Most tissues
High K_m	Low K_m
High V_m	Low V_m
Inhibited by glucose 6-phosphate	Not inhibited by glucose 6-phosphate
Induced by insulin	Unaffected by insulin or diet

9. In glycolysis

a. The phosphorylation of fructose 6-phosphate is catalysed by the enzyme phosphofructokinase

b. <u>One</u> molecule of glucose leads to the production of <u>one</u> molecule of pyruvate under aerobic conditions

c. There is a net gain of two molecules of ATP for each glucose molecule converted to lactate anaerobically

d. The reactions can only take place in the presence of oxygen

e. Aldolase catalyses the cleavage of a six-carbon sugar into two three-carbon molecules

10. Theme – glycolysis

Fill in the gaps in the passage below with selections from the following list

Options

A. Reduction
B. Four
C. Two
D. Isomerization
E. Erythrocytes
F. Spermatozoa
G. Facilitated diffusion
H. Passive diffusion
I. Oxidation
J. Phosphorylation

Glycolysis is a process that takes place in all cells of the body. It is important in ....$_1$, which lack mitochondria and use glycolysis as their only source of energy. Entry of one molecule of glucose into the glycolysis pathway leads to the production of ....$_2$ molecules of NADH, which undergo ....$_3$ by the electron transport chain in the production of ATP. Glucose enters cells by the process of ....$_4$ and is trapped within the cells by a ....$_5$ reaction in the first step of the pathway.

ATP, adenosine triphosphate; NAD⁺, oxidized form of nicotinamide adenine dinucleotide; NADH, reduced form of nicotinamide adenine dinucleotide; ADP, adenosine diphosphate

EXPLANATION: GLYCOLYSIS (ii)

Glucose enters cells by facilitated diffusion through specific transporter proteins. The first reaction of glycolysis, catalysed by hexokinase, phosphorylates glucose to glucose 6-phosphate. In the third reaction of the pathway, phosphofructokinase catalyses the transfer of another phosphate group using ATP, to give the product fructose 1,6-bisphosphate. The phosphorylated intermediates are trapped in the cytosol as they cannot diffuse across the cell membrane.

The next reaction, catalysed by aldolase, splits the hexose sugar to give dihydroxyacetone phosphate and glyceraldehyde phosphate (both triose sugars) so that eventually two molecules of pyruvate (or lactate) are produced from each glucose molecule.

Glycolysis has one oxidation reaction in which NAD^+ is converted to NADH, and this cofactor is oxidized by the electron transport chain if oxygen is available, or regenerated back to NAD^+ under anaerobic conditions by the conversion of pyruvate to lactate.

For cells that have no mitochondria, erythrocytes (red blood cells), for example, glycolysis provides the only source of ATP (two ATP per glucose).

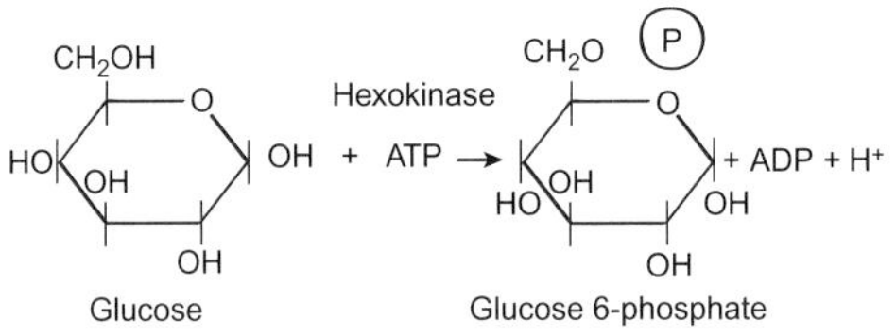

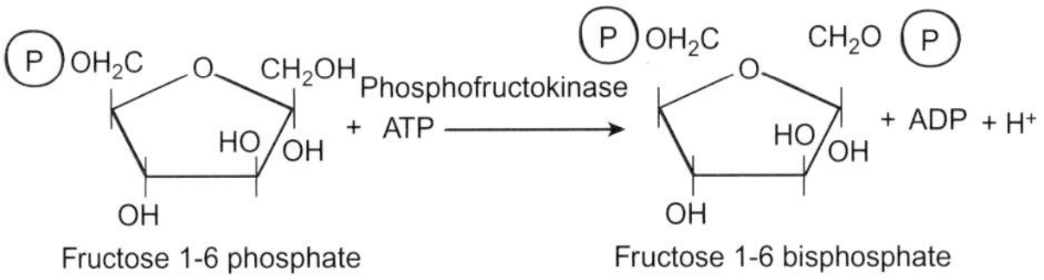

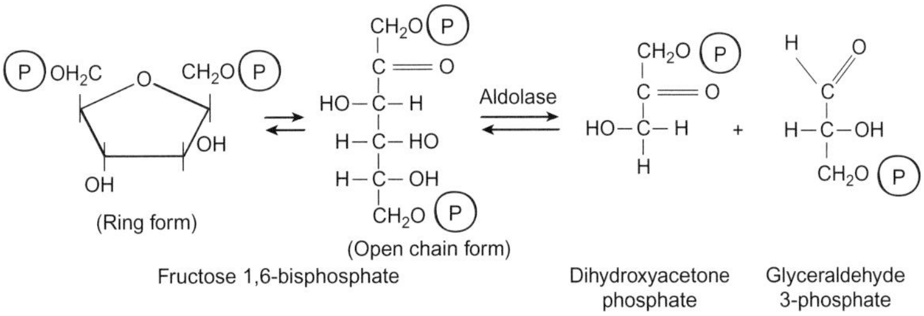

Glucose → Glucose 6-phosphate (Hexokinase, + ATP → + ADP + H⁺)

Fructose 1-6 phosphate → Fructose 1-6 bisphosphate (Phosphofructokinase, + ATP → + ADP + H⁺)

Fructose 1,6-bisphosphate (Ring form / Open chain form) → Dihydroxyacetone phosphate + Glyceraldehyde 3-phosphate (Aldolase)

Answers
9. T F T F T
10. 1 – E, 2 – C, 3 – I, 4 – G, 5 – J

11. In the regulation of glycolysis

    a. Hexokinase is inhibited by glucose 6-phosphate
    b. ATP inhibits the action of pyruvate kinase by an allosteric mechanism
    c. Citrate stimulates the action of phosphofructokinase
    d. ATP is an allosteric activator of phosphofructokinase
    e. ATP inhibits the action of aldolase

12. In the glycolysis pathway three of the steps are irreversible in vivo. Which enzymes catalyse these steps?

    a. Hexokinase
    b. Phosphofructokinase
    c. Pyruvate kinase
    d. Aldolase
    e. Glyceraldehyde 3-phosphate dehydrogenase

ATP, adenosine triphosphate; AMP, adenosine monophosphate

EXPLANATION: REGULATION OF GLYCOLYSIS

Hexokinase is inhibited by glucose 6-phosphate, the product of the reaction it catalyses. **Phosphofructokinase** is the key rate regulator of glycolysis. When ATP and citrate are present in high concentrations, there is reduced need for sugars to be sent through glycolysis and on to the citric acid cycle. **ATP and citrate allosterically inhibit phosphofructokinase**, and any consequent build up of glucose 6-phosphate can be used for glycogen synthesis. **Aldolase** is not a rate controlling step of glycolysis and is **not an allosteric enzyme**.

The **three physiologically irreversible steps** of glycolysis are catalysed by the enzymes **hexokinase, phosphofructokinase and pyruvate kinase**. If it were not for these steps, glucose could be generated from pyruvate by a simple reversal of the glycolytic reactions. Gluconeogenesis bypasses these steps by using different enzymes.

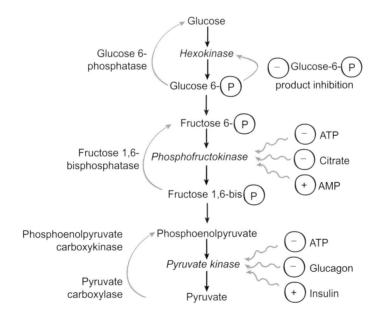

13. True or false? Glycogen

a. Makes up 6–8 per cent by weight of the adult liver
b. Acts as a fuel reserve during muscle contraction
c. Contains a backbone of glucose residues linked by α 1,6-linked bonds
d. Yields more ATP per g weight than fat
e. Liver stores are cleared within 4 hours of fasting

14. Regarding glycogen synthesis

a. One UTP and one ATP are required for each glucosyl residue formed
b. Uridine diphosphate glucose is formed from glucose and uridine triphosphate
c. Uridine diphosphate glucose donates glucosyl residues to the glycogen backbone
d. Branches are formed by α 1,4 linkage
e. Glycogen synthase forms α 1,4 linkages

15. Match the enzyme with the reaction

Options

A. Creation of branches on glycogen
B. Phosphorylation of glucose
C. Transfer of glucosyl residues from uridine diphosphate glucose to glycogen primer
D. Conversion of glucose 6-phosphate to glucose 1-phosphate
E. Formation of uridine diphosphate glucose from uridine triphosphate

1. Phosphoglucomutase
2. Uridine diphosphate glucose pyrophosphorylase
3. Glycogen synthase
4. Glucosyl 4:6 transferase
5. Hexokinase/glucokinase

ADP, adenosine diphosphate; ATP, adenosine triphosphate; UDP, uridine diphosphate; UTP, uridine triphosphate; PPi, pyrophosphate

EXPLANATION: GLYCOGEN – STRUCTURE AND SYNTHESIS

Glycogen is a **rapidly accessible** store of glucose used by the body in the absence of carbohydrate intake. It is found in the skeletal muscle and liver. Its stores are usually cleared within 18–24 hours of fasting. Glycogen is a **polymer of α-D glucose** residues linked by α **1,4 glycosidic bonds**.

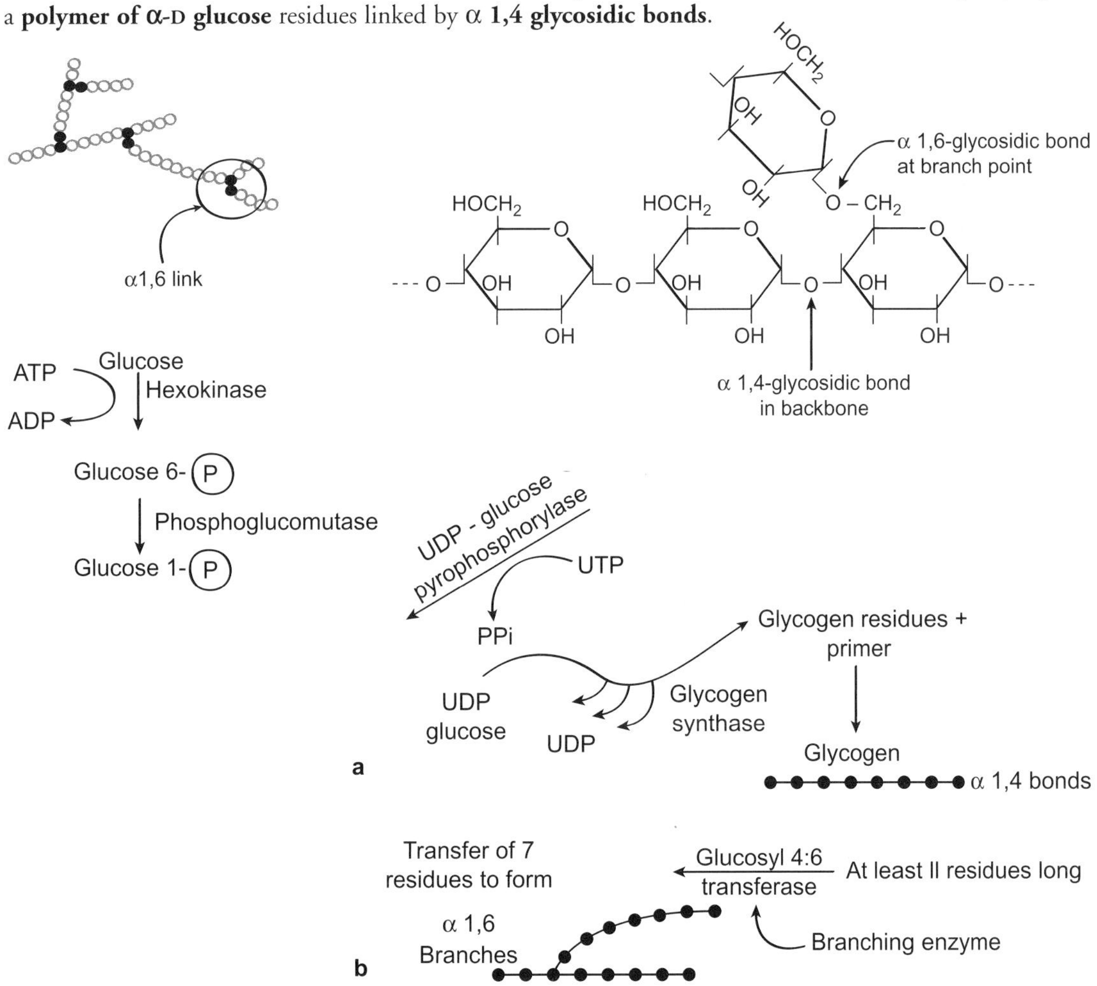

Glycogen synthesis occurs in the **cytosol** and **requires ATP** and UTP. **Glucose 6-phosphate** is converted to **UDP glucose** which acts as the glucosyl residue donor. Fragments of existing glycogen are the primer to which the α 1,4 linkages are added using the enzyme glycogen synthase. If there is no primer, a specific protein, glycogenin can act as an acceptor for the glucosyl residues.

Answers

13. T T F F F
14. T F T F T
15. 1 – D, 2 – E, 3 – C, 4 – A, 5 – B

16. Glycogen storage diseases

    a. Are autoimmune conditions
    b. Are always fatal
    c. Result from a defect in an enzyme for glycogen synthesis or degradation
    d. Can cause enlargement of the liver
    e. Affect all organs of the body

17. The following factors increase glycogen degradation in the liver

    a. Elevated plasma insulin levels
    b. Elevated glucagon levels
    c. Elevated adrenaline levels
    d. Elevated plasma glucose levels
    e. Increased intracellular cAMP levels

18. Explain the following terms with regard to the regulation of glycogen metabolism

    a. Covalent modification
    b. Allosteric activation

AMP, adenosine monophosphate; cAMP, cyclic adenosine monophosphate

EXPLANATION: DISORDERS OF GLYCOGEN STORAGE

Glycogen storage diseases are a group of **genetic** diseases that result from specific **enzyme defects**. Either glycogen is formed with abnormal structure or excessive amounts accumulate in specific tissues. Only a few of these inherited glycogen storage diseases are fatal, most of the conditions can be managed with special dietary regimes, or the avoidance of vigorous exercise.

Glycogenolysis (or glycogen degradation) requires two stages:

• **Shortening of glycogen chains** catalysed by **glycogen phosphorylase**
• **Removal of branches** catalysed by the enzyme **amylo-1,6-glucosidase**.

The regulation of glycogen degradation and synthesis is controlled by **two main mechanisms**. It is important to understand that **glycogen phosphorylase** (the key enzyme for degradation) and **glycogen synthase** (the key enzyme for synthesis) are controlled by the same hormonal signals, but these signals produce opposing actions for the two enzymes.

Only a few of these inherited glycogen storage diseases are fatal, most of the conditions can be managed with special dietary regimes, or the avoidance of vigorous exercise.

The two 'catabolic' hormones, **glucagon** and **adrenaline**, bind to G-protein linked membrane receptors in liver cells and activate **adenyl cyclase**. This causes an **increase in intracellular cAMP** which then activates **protein kinase A**. The protein kinase in turn causes a cascade of phosphorylation reactions on a range of intracellular enzymes. These reactions result in the phosphorylation and **inactivation of glycogen synthase** to inhibit glycogen synthesis, and **activation of glycogen phosphorylase** to promote glycogen breakdown to glucose. **Insulin has the opposite affect to glucagon** and adrenaline, and **promotes glycogen synthesis** and storage.

This phosphorylation/dephosphorylation mechanism of control is known as **covalent modification (18a)**.

Another mechanism of control is **allosteric activation**, whereby glycogen phosphorylase and glycogen synthase respond to levels of certain small metabolites **(18b)**. In the muscle Ca^{2+} and AMP initiate glycogen degradation. In the liver, glucose inhibits degradation, whereas glucose 6-phosphate activates glycogen synthesis.

Answers

16. F F T T F
17. F T T F T
18. See explanation

19. True or false? The citric acid cycle

a. Takes place in the cytosol
b. Produces NADH
c. Is the main source of energy in erythrocytes
d. Can take place in anaerobic conditions
e. Includes a precursor of porphyrin synthesis

20. Theme – the citric acid cycle

Fill in the gaps in the following passage by selecting from the list below

Options

A. Aspartate
B. Four
C. Three
D. Two
E. Five

F. Nucleus
G. Albumin
H. Cytosol
I. Mitochondria
J. Porphyrins/heme

The citric acid cycle is a metabolic pathway that oxidizes acetyl CoA, producing ...₁... molecules of CO_2. The citric acid cycle takes place in the ...₂... . The citric acid cycle produces ...₃... molecules of NADH and one molecule of $FADH_2$ per cycle, which go on to be oxidized by the electron transport chain. The cycle also produces precursors for other biosynthetic pathways, for example malate can enter gluconeogenesis, and ...₄... is synthesized from succinyl CoA.

21. True or false? The process of pyruvate decarboxylation by the pyruvate dehydrogenase complex produces

a. NADH
b. ATP
c. CO_2
d. Acetyl CoA
e. Lactate

ATP, adenosine triphosphate; NADH, reduced form of nicotinamide adenine dinucleotide; TCA, tricarboxylic acid; $FADH_2$, reduced form of flavine adenine dinucleotide; FAD, flavine adenine dinucleotide; NAD^+, oxidized form of nicotinamide adenine dinucleotide; GTP, guanosine triphosphate

EXPLANATION: THE CITRIC ACID CYCLE

The **citric acid cycle** (also known as the **tricarboxylic acid cycle**, **TCA cycle**, **Krebs cycle**) oxidizes acetyl CoA in **mitochondria**. The cycle produces CO_2, **NADH and FADH$_2$**. The NADH and FADH$_2$ enter oxidative phosphorylation, where they are oxidized to NAD^+ and FAD, ready to be used in the citric acid cycle again. The citric acid cycle is also important in some biosynthetic processes such as **lipid synthesis, amino acid synthesis, porphyrin synthesis** and **gluconeogenesis**.

The citric acid cycle takes place entirely within the **mitochondrial matrix**. Three of the reactions in the cycle **generate NADH**: (1) the decarboxylation of isocitrate, (2) the decarboxylation of α-ketoglutarate and (3) the oxidation of malate. **Erythrocytes do not utilize the citric acid cycle** as an energy source as they have no mitochondria. None of the reactions of the citric acid cycle requires the presence of molecular oxygen. However, the NAD^+ required by three of the reactions **is regenerated by oxidative phosphorylation**; in anaerobic conditions NAD^+ stores are depleted and the citric acid cycle stops. **Succinyl CoA** is used in the production of porphyrins.

The **citric acid cycle** does not directly produce ATP. One cycle produces **three molecules of NADH, one of GTP, one of FADH$_2$ and two of CO$_2$**. The citric acid cycle can **only take place in aerobic conditions** – while molecular O_2 is not required by any of the reactions in the cycle, the NAD^+ and FAD are generated by oxidative phosphorylation, and in the absence of O_2 mitochondrial stores of these carrier molecules soon run out and the cycle ceases.

The **pyruvate dehydrogenase** complex comprises three enzymes – **pyruvate decarboxylase, lipoamide transacetylase** and **dihydrolipoyl dehydrogenase**. In eukaryotes it is located in the mitochondrial matrix. **Pyruvate** is decarboxylated to produce **NADH, acetyl CoA** and **CO$_2$**.

Answers

19. F T F F T
20. 1 – D, 2 – I, 3 – C, 4 – J
21. T F T T F

22. **Points 1–5 in the diagram below indicate compounds in the citric acid cycle. Select the correct label for each point from the following list**

Options

A. Succinyl CoA
B. Isocitrate
C. Oxaloacetate
D. Succinate
E. Malate
F. Fumarate
G. Citrate
H. Pyruvate
I. α-Ketoglutarate
J. Lactate

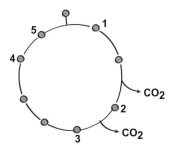

23. **Match the following important intermediates of the citric acid cycle with the actions below**

A. Lactate
B. α-Ketoglutarate
C. Fumarate
D. Succinate
E. Oxaloacetate

F. Malate
G. Succinyl CoA
H. Acetyl CoA
I. Isocitrate
J. Pyruvate

1. The action of ATP-citrate lyase on citrate produces this compound, which may be used in fatty acid synthesis
2. Condensation of this compound with glycine in mitochondria is the first step in haem synthesis
3. This four carbon compound is regenerated by each complete turn of the citric acid cycle
4. Transfer of the amino group of alanine to this compound by the enzyme alanine aminotransferase produces glutamate
5. In the process of gluconeogenesis, this compound may be converted to phosphoenolpyruvate by the action of phosphoenolpyruvate-carboxykinase

---

NADH, reduced form of nicotinamide adenine dinucleotide; FADH$_2$, reduced form of flavine adenine dinucleotide; TCA, tricarboxylic acid; ATP, adenosine triphosphate; FA, fatty acid

EXPLANATION: METABOLIC IMPORTANCE OF CITRIC ACID CYCLE

The biosynthetic roles of glycolysis and the TCA cycle are shown in the diagram below.

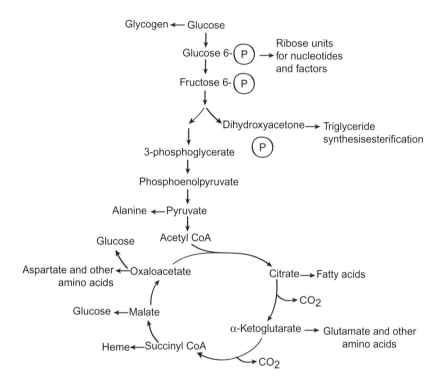

The reaction that catalyses the synthesis of citrate in the citric acid cycle is:

$$\text{Oxaloacetate (+ } H_2O) + \text{Acetyl CoA} \rightarrow \text{Citrate (+ CoA)}$$

NADH and $FADH_2$ are oxidized in the electron transport chain. Each cycle of the citric acid cycle produces three molecules of NADH and one molecule of $FADH_2$.

Oxaloacetate and α-keto glutarate (also known as 2-oxoglutarate) can be converted to aspartate and glutamate by specific aminotransferase enzymes. Citrate can be used to generate acetyl CoA for FA synthesis in the cytosol, by the action of citrate lyase.

Answers
22. 1 – G, 2 – I, 3 – A, 4 – E, 5 – C
23. 1 – H, 2 – G, 3 – E, 4 – B, 5 – E

24. True or false? In oxidative phosphorylation

a. H_2O is produced from the oxidation of NADH and $FADH_2$
b. The presence of molecular oxygen is not required
c. ATP synthase is composed of a H^+ carrier (F_0 subunit) and a motor protein (F_1 subunit)
d. Active pumping of protons by electron transport chain proteins requires ATP
e. The electron transport chain proteins lie on the inner mitochondrial membrane

25. Theme – oxidative phosphorylation. Fill in the gaps in the passage below with terms from the following list

Options

A. ATP
C. Ubiquinone
E. ADP
G. Outer
I. H^+

B. $FADH_2$
D. NADPH
F. Inner
H. Rotenone
J. Na^+

In the process of oxidative phosphorylation, electrons are eventually transferred to oxygen molecules from NADH and ....1. The electron transfer chain is composed of a series of membrane proteins located on the ....2 mitochondrial membrane. The energy released as the electrons are passed to lower energy states is coupled to the pumping of ....3 ions across the membrane. Electrons are ferried between proteins of the electron transport chain by cytochrome c and ....4 molecules. The ion gradient created by the electron transport chain proteins is used to drive synthesis of ....5.

26. True of false? The following drugs and toxins disrupt the process of oxidative phosphorylation by acting as inhibitors or uncouplers

a. Penicillin
b. Adrenaline
c. 2,4-Dinitrophenol
d. Paracetamol
e. Cyanide

ADP, adenosine diphosphate; ATP, adenosine triphosphate; NADH, reduced form of nicotinamide adenine dinucleotide; NADPH, reduced form of nicotinamide adenine dinucleotide phosphate; $FADH_2$, reduced form of flavine adenine dinucleotide; PL, inorganic phosphate

EXPLANATION: OXIDATIVE PHOSPHORYLATION

Electrons donated by NADH and $FADH_2$ are passed along the **electron transport chain proteins**, which are embedded in the **inner mitochondrial membrane**. Electrons move to lower energy states at each stage, and it is the energy released by this process that is coupled to the pumping of protons across the membrane. At the last electron transport chain protein, the cytochrome oxidase complex, two electrons combine with two protons and molecular oxygen to produce water.

ATP synthase is an 'energy coupling' protein, composed of a H^+ carrier (the F_0 subunit) that is located in the inner mitochondrial membrane, and a motor protein (the F_1 subunit). The F_1 subunit generates ATP from Pi and ADP, a process that is driven by the flow of H^+ ions through the F_0 subunit, down their concentration gradient from the intermembrane space to the matrix compartment of the mitochondria.

2,4-Dinitrophenol is a lipophilic chemical which can penetrate the lipid bilayers of the mitochondrial membranes and 'carry' H^+ ions across in either direction. Re-entry of proteins (H^- ions) across the membrane by any process other than through the ATP synthase mechanism (the F_0–F_1 channel protein) will interfere with the generation of the H^+ gradient, and ATP synthesis will decrease, even though the oxidation of NADH and $FADH_2$ continues. This results in the 'uncoupling' of ATP synthesis from the metabolism of carbohydrates and fats, and their chemical energy will be wasted as heat.

It has been suggested by some experimental data that hormones such as thyroxine may increase the rate of intermediary metabolism by an 'uncoupling' effect on mitochondrial function, but adrenaline has no such affect. Aspirin and the 'recreational drug'. Ecstasy may also have an 'uncoupling effect' on mitochondrial function at high doses. Paracetamol and penicillin do not have any known effects on oxidative phosphorylation.

Cyanide inhibits the action of one of the electron transfer chain proteins, but proton transport remains coupled to ATP production. Other inhibitors of oxidative phosphorylation are rotenone, amytal and carbon monoxide.

Answers
24. T F T F T
25. 1 – B, 2 – F, 3 – I, 4 – C, 5 – A
26. F F T F T

27. Sources for gluconeogenesis include

a. Lactate
b. Acetyl CoA
c. Leucine
d. Glycerol
e. Aspartate

28. Gluconeogenesis in the liver is stimulated by increases in

a. Glucagon
b. Intracellular cAMP
c. Glucocorticoids
d. Intracellular ATP
e. Insulin

29. Which of the following are important bypass reactions in gluconeogenesis?

a. Carboxylation of pyruvate to oxaloacetate
b. Conversion of fructose 6-phosphate to glucose 6-phosphate
c. Conversion of oxaloacetate to phosphoenolpyruvate
d. Dephosphorylation of fructose 1,6-bisphosphate
e. Dephosphorylation of glucose 6-phosphate

ATP, adenosine triphosphate; TAG, triacylglycerol; FA, fatty acids; TCA, tricarboxylic acid; cAMP, cyclic adenosine monophosphate

EXPLANATION: GLUCONEOGENESIS (i)

When hepatic **glycogen** stores are depleted in the early stages of fasting, glucose can be formed from precursors by **gluconeogenesis** in the **liver** and also the **kidney**.

Sources for gluconeogenesis include all the **intermediates** of glycolysis and the TCA cycle, **glycerol** from the hydrolysis of TAGs, and **lactate**. All the **amino acids** except leucine, lysine, phenylalanine, tyrosine and isoleucine are glucogenic. They are converted to α-ketoacids which can be converted to **oxaloacetate** and then to phosphoenolpyruvate, which is an intermediate of the gluconeogenic pathway. FA cannot be used for gluconeogenesis. FAs are broken down by β-oxidation which results in acetyl CoA production, and this cannot be converted into any three-carbon or four-carbon compounds in the human liver, as the pyruvate dehydrogenase reaction is irreversible.

Glucagon stimulates gluconeogenesis by several mechanisms. Firstly, the hormone mobilizes substrates for the pathway by releasing glycerol from triglycerides (TAGs) by the action of adipose tissue lipase. Secondly, glucagon elevates intracellular levels of cAMP which then stimulates protein kinase A to its active form. This phosphorylates pyruvate kinase to its inactive form. As a result less pyruvate is formed from phosphoenolpyruvate and thus more phosphoenolpyruvate is diverted into the gluconeogenic pathway.

Lastly, both glucagon and the glucocorticoid hormones, such as cortisol increase the levels of the glucogenic 'bypass' enzymes such as fructose 1,6-bisphosphatase and glucose 6-phosphatase, and also the levels of the transaminase enzymes which release the carbon skeletons from the glucogenic amino acids.

Insulin has the opposite effect to glucagon in decreasing the levels of the gluconeogenic 'bypass' enzymes.

Gluconeogenesis uses seven of the **reversible** reactions of glycolysis in the synthesis of glucose from pyruvate or lactate. However, three of the reactions of glycolysis are **irreversible**. Therefore these steps have to be bypassed using four reactions unique to gluconeogenesis. See page 26 for the diagram of the pathway of glycolysis/gluconeogenesis.

Answers

27. T F F T T
28. T T T F F
29. T F T T T

30. True or false? With regard to gluconeogenesis

a. All the steps of gluconeogenesis are those of glycolysis in reverse
b. It occurs chiefly in the liver and kidneys
c. The fatty acid portion of triglycerides can be converted to glucose
d. The glycerol portion of triglycerides can be converted to glucose
e. The reaction catalysed by pyruvate carboxylase takes place in the cytosol

31. Pyruvate carboxylation

a. In the gluconeogenesis pathway, describe the reaction for the conversion of pyruvate to phosphoenolpyruvate, including the enzymes and cofactors
b. What is the biological importance of the reaction catalysed by pyruvate carboxylase in the citric acid cycle?

32. Theme – gluconeogenesis

Complete the paragraph below using terms from the following list

Options

A. Two	**B.** One
C. Four	**D.** Three
E. Fatty acids	**F.** Mitochondria
G. Adipose	**H.** Liver
I. Skeletal muscle	**J.** Glycerol
K. Acetyl CoA	**L.** Cytosol
M. Endoplasmic reticulum	**N.** Golgi apparatus

Blood glucose levels must be tightly controlled. In starvation or prolonged exercise, dietary glucose and glycogen stores may become exhausted. In these situations, blood glucose levels are maintained by the process of gluconeogenesis. Gluconeogenesis produces glucose from ...., lactate and amino acids. Gluconeogenesis takes place in .... cells and to a lesser extent in the kidneys. The carboxylation of pyruvate to produce oxaloacetate takes place in the .... but all the other reactions occur in the .... Gluconeogenesis is not a straightforward reversal of the glycolysis pathway as there are .... irreversible steps in glycolysis that must be bypassed.

FA, fatty acid; GDP, guanosine diphosphate; GTP, guanosine triphosphate; MDH, malate dehydrogenase; TAG, triacylglycerol; FFA, free fatty acid; ATP, adenosine triphosphate

EXPLANATION: GLUCONEOGENESIS (ii)

Gluconeogenesis is not a straightforward reversal of glycolysis as there are three irreversible steps in glycolysis that must be bypassed. The conversion of phosphoenolpyruvate to pyruvate is one of these irreversible steps.

In order to progress from pyruvate to glucose, pyruvate is first carboxylated in mitochondria to form oxaloacetate. The action of malate dehydrogenase converts oxaloacetate to malate, which is able to leave the mitochondria and enter the cytosol where the reverse reaction regenerates oxaloacetate. The enzyme phosphoenolpyruvate carboxykinase then catalyses the phosphorylation and decarboxylation of oxaloacetate to form phosphoenolpyruvate (31a).

Pyruvate carboxylase catalyses the conversion of pyruvate to oxaloacetate using ATP and CO_2. This is an important reaction both for gluconeogenesis (to bypass the pyruvate kinase reaction) and also for the normal function of the citric acid cycle. For the citric acid cycle to begin, one molecule each of oxaloacetate and acetyl CoA is required. If there is a shortage of oxaloacetate, the balance is restored by the action of pyruvate carboxylase. If, for example, oxaloacetate has been removed from the cycle to enter the amino acid synthesis pathways, it can simply be regenerated from pyruvate (31b).

The main site of gluconeogenesis is the liver, and to a lesser extent the kidneys. The FA portions of triglycerides are converted to acetyl CoA in mitochondria and enter the citric acid cycle. The glycerol portion of triglyceride is converted to glycerol 3-phosphate and may be converted to glucose by gluconeogenesis.

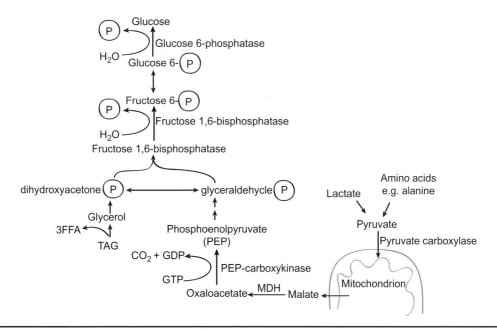

Answers

30. F T F T F
31. See explanation
32. 1 – J, 2 – H, 3 – F, 4 – L, 5 – D

EXPLANATION: GLUCOSE METABOLISM (CONT.)

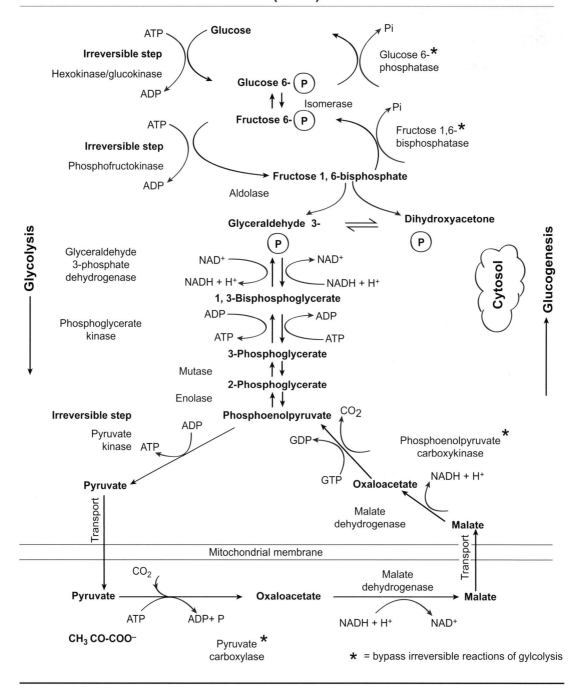

ATP, adenosine triphosphate; ADP, adenosine diphosphate; NAD⁺, oxidized form of nicotinamide adenine dinucleotide; NADH, reduced form of nicotinamide adenine dinucleotide; GDP, guanosine diphosphate; GTP, guanosine triphosphate; Pi, inorganic phosphate

SECTION 2
LIPID AND AMINO ACID METABOLISM

- FATTY ACIDS (i)   28
- FATTY ACIDS (ii)   30
- FATTY ACID OXIDATION   32
- FATTY ACID SYNTHESIS   34
- LIPID SYNTHESIS   36
- CHOLESTEROL   38
- LIPID TRANSPORT   40
- PLASMA LIPOPROTEINS   42
- KETONE BODY SYNTHESIS   44
- PROTEIN TURNOVER   46
- AMINO ACID METABOLISM   48
- UREA CYCLE   50
- DIETARY ASPECTS OF AMINO ACIDS   52

LIPID METABOLISM AND AMINO ACID METABOLISM

1. True or false? Fatty acids

a. Are amphipathic
b. Are carried in the bloodstream bound to albumin
c. Are saturated if they have one or more double bonds
d. Double bonds are usually in the *trans*-configuration
e. Can be synthesized in the lactating mammary glands

2. Linoleic acid

a. Has 18 carbon atoms in its chain
b. Is unsaturated
c. Is an ω-6 fatty acid
d. Is an essential fatty acid
e. May be a precursor to arachidonic acid

3. Essential fatty acids

a. Can be synthesized by vertebrates
b. Have double bonds at ω-9
c. Are found in fish oils
d. May be used as substrates for gluconeogenesis
e. Are required for synthesis of eicosanoids

FA, fatty acid

EXPLANATION: FATTY ACIDS (i)

Fatty acids (FAs) have a **-COOH group** on the end of their hydrocarbon chain which ionizes at physiologi-cal pH to give them a hydrophilic region as well as a hydrophobic region (they are amphipathic). Long-chain FAs are predominantly hydrophobic and thus require a carrier in circulation – **albumin**. Saturated FAs have no double bonds. Double bonds can be inserted by desaturating enzymes at positions up to nine carbon atoms from the methyl end, in which case they become unsaturated. **Monounsaturated** implies just one double bond; **polyunsaturated** implies two, three or four double bonds.

Name	Carbon atoms	Double bonds	Formula
Saturated			
Butyric acid	4	0	$CH_3-CH_2-CH_2-COOH$
Palmitic acid	16	0	$CH_3-(CH_2)_{14}-COOH$
Stearic acid	18	0	$CH_3-(CH_2)_{16}-COOH$
Unsaturated			
Linoleic acid	18	2	$CH_3-(CH_2)_4-CH=CH-CH_2-CH=CH-(CH_2)_7-COOH$

$$CH_3\underset{\underset{\omega}{(18)}}{-}(CH_2)_4-CH=CH-CH_2-CH\underset{(12)}{=}CH\underset{(9)}{-}(CH_2)_7\underset{(1)\,or\,\alpha}{-}COOH$$

Linoleic acid 18:2 has two carbon double bonds. It is referred to as an **omega-6 FA** because the closest double bond to the terminal ω carbon atom is six carbon atoms from the end of the chain.

Structure of linolenic acid

Cis-configuration
double bond

COOH

Two FAs are essential in humans: **linoleic acid** and **linolenic acid**. They are both polyunsaturated FAs, and they both have double bonds at ω6. They must be taken in the diet since they cannot be synthesized. Most other polyunsaturated FAs (such as arachidonic acid $C_{22:4}$) can be made to some extent from these two 'parent' FAs. It is possible that arachidonic acid is essential in the diet of young children, or in certain other conditions that result in high demand for the polyunsaturated FAs. Polyunsaturated FAs are required for maintenance of fluidity of the cell membranes and synthesis of eicosanoids. See page 83 for the trans double bonds.

Answers
1. T T F F T
2. T T T T T
3. F F T F T

4. Which of the following are essential dietary fatty acids?

    a. Oleic acid
    b. Palmitic acid
    c. Linoleic acid
    d. Stearic acid
    e. Linolenic acid

5. Concerning fats

    a. Triglycerides are composed of three fatty acid chains bound to glycine
    b. Metabolism of long chain fatty acids requires carnitine for transfer into the mitochondria
    c. Cholesterol is the precursor for the synthesis of all the steroid hormones
    d. Fatty acids synthesized in the body are all even-numbered in terms of the carbon atom chain (C_{16}, C_{18}, C_{20} etc)
    e. Fatty acids can be broken down completely in the body to CO_2 and H_2O

6. Which of the following are saturated fatty acids?

    a. Stearic acid
    b. Oleic acid
    c. Arachidonic acid
    d. Linoleic acid
    e. Palmitic acid

7. The following cells can utilize fatty acids as fuels

    a. Brain neurons
    b. Liver cells
    c. Erythrocytes
    d. Renal cells
    e. Muscle cells

FA, fatty acid

EXPLANATION: FATTY ACIDS (ii)

Although FAs can be synthesized in the body, when fed a totally fat-free diet animals fail to thrive unless provided with the three essential FAs – linolenic, linoleic and arachidonic acid. It is believed that humans have a similar dependence on an exogenous source of these three FAs and they are therefore known as the essential FAs. Arachidonic can be made to a certain extent in adults from linoleic acid, and may only be essential in children.

Triglycerides are made up of three FAs attached to one molecule of glycerol. Short-chain FAs may cross the inner mitochondrial membrane. Carnitine is not an FA, but is part of the shuttle mechanism that passes acyl CoA molecules into mitochondria. FAs are broken down by β-oxidation to form acetyl CoA.

Arachidonic acid is a 20-carbon lipid found in phospholipid membranes. It is a precursor for many important compounds including prostaglandins and thromboxane A_2. Cholesterol is an important component of plasma membranes and is also a precursor to the steroid hormones such as cortisol and testosterone.

FA metabolism is oxidative, and occurs in two stages, firstly β-oxidation to acetyl CoA, which is then oxidized in the citric acid cycle to CO_2 and H_2O. Both pathways occur in mitochondria. Most tissues are able to produce acetyl CoA from FAs, and the process is particularly important in liver and muscle cells. Certain cells are unable to oxidize FAs as they either do not contain the necessary enzymes (brain, adrenal medulla) or they do not have mitochondria (erythrocytes).

Biologically important FAs in human tissues are:

Palmitic acid	C16:0
Stearic acid	C18:0
Oleic acid	C18:1
Linoleic acid	C18:2
γ-Linolenic acid	C18:3
Arachidonic acid	C20:4

Answers

4. F F T F T
5. F T T T T
6. T F F F T
7. F T F T T

8. Preparation of fats for oxidation. Fill in the gaps in the passage below using terms from the following list

A. Citrate

C. Carnitine

E. Cholesterol

G. Dehydrogenation

I. Phosphorylation

K. Malonyl CoA

M. Dihydroxyacetone phosphate

B. Malate-aspartate

D. Phosphoenolpyruvate

F. Glycine

H. Hydrolysis

J. Coenzyme A

L. Glycerol

N. 1,3-Phosphglyceric acid

The triglycerides stored in adipose cells are a major energy store. Utilization of lipids in generating ATP begins with .... of triglycerides, producing three fatty acid chains and one molecule of ...., which can enter the glycolysis pathway by conversion to .... The free fatty acids are bound to albumin and transported in the blood to their target tissues. After uptake by target cells a free fatty acid is attached to a molecule of .... and transported into mitochondria by the .... shuttle.

9. β-Oxidation of fatty acids

a. Takes place in the cytosol

b. Produces $FADH_2$

c. Produces GTP

d. Produces NADH

e. Produces acetyl CoA

10. True or false? The process of β-oxidation of fatty acids

a. Is a source of acetyl CoA

b. Is a source of glucose

c. Removes one carbon from the fatty acid chain at each pass

d. Requires ATP at the activation stage

e. Is stimulated by insulin

FA, fatty acid; $FADH_2$, reduced form of flavine adenine dinucleotide; GTP, guanosine triphosphate; NADH, reduced form of nicotinamide adenine dinucleotide; ATP, adenosine triphosphate; NAD^+, oxidized form of nicotinamide adenine dinucleotide; FAD, flavine adenine dinucleotide; TAG, triacylglycerol

EXPLANATION: FATTY ACID OXIDATION

FAs are oxidized by the β-oxidation pathway which breaks down the FA chin, two carbon atoms at a time to give **acetyl CoA**. The first enzyme reaction takes place in the cytosol and results in a long chain FA being converted to its CoA ester by an **ATP-dependent activating enzyme**. **The transfer of the fatty acyl CoA ester into the mitochondria** matrix occurs next and requires **carnitine**.

The sequence of four enzyme reactions shown in the diagram below results in the removal of two pairs of hydrogen atoms from the fatty acyl CoA molecule which are passed to the cofactors NAD^+ and FAD which become **reduced to NADH and $FADH_2$**. As these reactions occur in the mitochondria, it is easy for the cofactors to be rapidly **reoxidized by the electron transport process** (the cytochrome chain) and this results in **ATP synthesis**. **A molecule of acetyl CoA is produced per turn of the β-oxidation spiral**. This acetyl CoA can be further metabolized to CO_2, but cannot be used as a source of intermediates for glucose synthesis by gluconeogenesis.

The molecules of acetyl CoA produced by β-oxidation then enter the citric acid cycle and are metabolized to CO_2 and H_2O. Thus a further 10 (or 12) ATP molecules may be synthesized for each acetyl CoA produced. The process is activated by adrenaline and glucagon which both increase the availability of FAs from the TAG stores in adipose tissue. **Insulin has the effect of decreasing FA oxidation** and **promoting fat synthesis**.

The figure below shows the β-oxidation pathway of fatty acid oxidation.

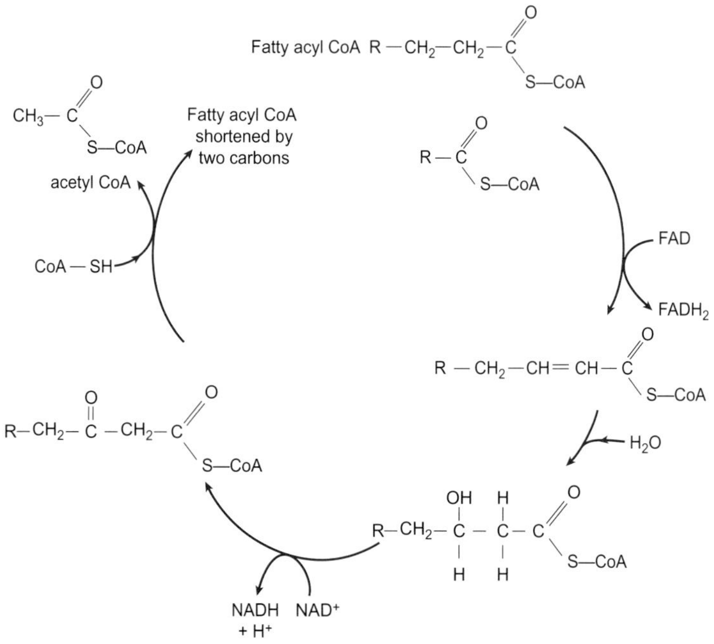

Answers

8. 1 – H, 2 – L, 3 – M, 4 – J, 5 – C
9. F T F T T
10. T F F T F

11. Fatty acid synthesis

a. Occurs in the liver cytosol
b. Requires a supply of acetyl CoA from the mitochondria
c. Requires a high concentration of citrate in the mitochondria
d. Involves carboxylation of acetyl CoA to malonyl CoA
e. Is stimulated by palmitoyl CoA

12. Fatty acid synthase

a. Is a multi-enzyme complex
b. Condenses acetyl CoA and malonyl CoA to form a four-carbon keto intermediate
c. Produces saturated fatty acids
d. Produces two molecules of NADPH
e. Generates palmitate as the final product

13. Concerning fatty acid synthesis

a. The process is inhibited by insulin
b. Each cycle adds a two-carbon unit to the chain
c. The process is endergonic (energy dependent)
d. NADPH is supplied by the hexose monophosphate pathway
e. Malonyl CoA is converted to acetyl CoA in the first step of the pathway

14. Use words from the following list of options to fill in the gaps in the paragraph about lipogenesis below

Options

A. Four	B. Oxaloacetate	C. Citrate	D. Enoyl CoA
E. Malonyl CoA	F. Mitochondria	G. Cytosol	H. Blood
I. Nucleus	J. Two		

Synthesis of fatty acids takes place in the ......$_1$..., but depends on a supply of acetyl CoA from the ......$_2$.... In order to move between the two compartments, acetyl-CoA is converted to ......$_3$.... To begin synthesis of a new fatty acid, both acetyl CoA and ......$_4$.... are attached to fatty acid synthase and are then combined by a sequence of reactions to form a short-chain fatty acid. The cycle can be repeated, combining acetyl CoA with the fatty acid formed in the last cycle, with ......$_5$.... carbons being added to the chain with each pass.

FA, fatty acid; NADPH, reduced form of nicotinamide adenine dinucleotide phosphate; TAG, triacylglycerol; ATP, adenosine triphosphate

EXPLANATION: FATTY ACID SYNTHESIS

FA synthesis takes place in the **liver**, **lactating mammary glands**, **adipose tissue** and the **kidney**. Excess **protein** and **carbohydrate** can be converted to FAs and stored as **TAG**.

The first step is the formation of **malonyl CoA** from **acetyl CoA**. The CoA part of the acetyl CoA cannot cross the **mitochondrial membrane** to the **cytosol** where FA synthesis takes place. However, acetyl CoA and oxaloacetate condense to form citrate in the mitochondria, which can then cross to the cytosol. Citrate is only translocated across the membrane when the concentration is high in the mitochondria. Citrate is then cleaved to generate acetyl CoA in the cytosol.

FA synthase is a multi-enzyme complex. Each monomer has seven different enzymic activities. **Malonyl CoA** and **acetyl CoA** bind to the complex and undergo a series of reactions to give a four-carbon compound. The cycle of reactions is repeated seven times, incorporating two C atoms from malonyl CoA each time until a 16-carbon chain – palmitate – is formed.

Sources of **NADPH** required for the reaction are:

* The hexose monophosphate pathway
* The cytosolic conversion of malate to pyruvate

The process of FA synthesis by the cytosolic multi-enzyme pathway produces even numbered fully saturated FAs, with palmitic acid as the main end product. Palmitoyl CoA acts as a feedback inhibitor at the first step of the pathway, acetyl CoA carboxylase. As this enzyme requires ATP, the overall process of FA synthesis is energy dependent. The whole process is stimulated by insulin and occurs in the fed state after a high calorie meal. Longer chain FAs and monounsaturated FAs can be synthesized by specific elongating and 'desaturating' enzymes located on the endoplasmic reticulum of liver cells.

Answers

11. T T T T F
12. T T T F T
13. F T T T F
14. 1 – G, 2 – F, 3 – C, 4 – E, 5 – J

15. The acetyl CoA used in fatty acid synthesis can come from

a. The reaction catalysed by pyruvate dehydrogenase
b. The reaction catalysed by enoyl CoA hydratase
c. The degradation of purely glycogenic amino acids
d. The degradation of purely ketogenic amino acids
e. The degradation of cholesterol

16. True or false? Triacyglycerols

a. Are only synthesized in the liver
b. Are highly hydrophilic
c. Are synthesized on stimulation by insulin
d. Require glycerol phosphate for their synthesis
e. Usually carry a saturated fatty acid on carbon atom 1

17. Biologically important lipids

a. List three examples of biologically important lipids
b. Use a sketch diagram to show the arrangement of lipids in: (1) a mixed micelle, (2) the plasma membrane and (3) a lipoprotein complex

TAG, triacylglycerol; FA, fatty acid

EXPLANATION: LIPID SYNTHESIS

While FAs cannot be converted to carbohydrates in the body, conversion of carbohydrates to triglyceride fats is very important in the fed state. FA synthesis occurs in the cytosol. The FA synthase complex generates FA from acetyl CoA precursors. The first step of the pathway is the carboxylation of acetyl CoA to form malonyl CoA.

Pyruvate dehydrogenase produces acetyl CoA which can be used in synthesis of FAs. Enoyl CoA hydratase is an enzyme of the β-oxidation pathway and does not produce acetyl CoA. The three glycogenic amino acids are alanine, serine and glycine; they cannot be directly converted to acetyl CoA. The ketogenic amino acid isoleucine may be converted directly to acetyl CoA. Cholesterol is synthesized from acetyl CoA. However, cholesterol cannot be degraded in the body and is disposed of by excretion in bile.

TAGs consist of **three molecules of FAs esterified to a molecule of glycerol**. They are stored in **adipose tissue** and the **liver**, as well as circulating in the **blood**. Glycerol phosphate is the initial acceptor of FAs in TAG synthesis. Glycerol is phosphorylated for this initial step by glycerol kinase in the liver, but adipose tissue relies on glycolysis for a supply of glycerol phosphate.

There are three groups of biologically important lipids **(17a)**: **TAGs** – major energy reserve, **phospholipids** – contain a phosphate group esterified to another compound, and **steroids** – including cholesterol, parent compound of all steroids. For the structure of TAG see page 83.

Phospholipids generally arrange themselves such that hydrophobic groups are not in contact with fluid while hydrophilic groups are. The diagram below shows three ways in which they may group **(17b)**.

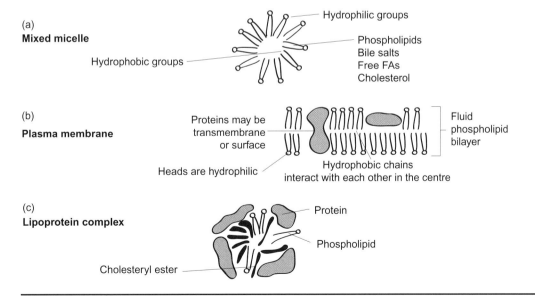

(a)
Mixed micelle

Hydrophilic groups

Hydrophobic groups

Phospholipids
Bile salts
Free FAs
Cholesterol

(b)
Plasma membrane

Proteins may be transmembrane or surface

Heads are hydrophilic

Hydrophobic chains interact with each other in the centre

Fluid phospholipid bilayer

(c)
Lipoprotein complex

Protein

Phospholipid

Cholesteryl ester

Answers
15. T F T T F
16. F F T T T
17. See explanation and diagram

18. Cholesterol

   a. Is highly hydrophobic
   b. Is the major sterol in animal tissues
   c. Is synthesized in the gall bladder
   d. Regulates the pathway for its own synthesis
   e. Is essential in the diet

19. True or false? HMG CoA reductase

   a. Is the rate limiting step of cholesterol synthesis
   b. Is inhibited by insulin
   c. Is located on the outer mitochondrial membrane
   d. Is inhibited by glucagon
   e. Is the target enzyme for the statin drugs

20. With reference to the biological functions of cholesterol

   a. It is the precursor for all the steroid hormones
   b. It has a major influence on the fluidity of the cell plasma membrane
   c. It is transported from the liver to peripheral tissues in the form of high density lipoprotein complexes
   d. It is converted into bile salts for excretion
   e. It can act as an alternative fuel for tissue metabolism during starvation

---

HMG CoA, 3-hydroxy-3-methylglutaryl CoA; NADPH, reduced form of nicotinamide adenine dinucleotide phosphate; ATP, adenosine triphosphate; LDL, low density lipoprotein

EXPLANATION: CHOLESTEROL

Cholesterol is the **major sterol in the body** and acts as both an **important component of cell membranes** (**controlling the fluidity** of the **phospholipid bilayer**) and also as the **precursor for the synthesis of the steroid hormones**. Cholesterol can be obtained from the diet in meat and dairy products, but is synthesized mainly in the liver, and then transported to other tissues of the body as LDL complexes in the plasma. All tissues are capable of cholesterol synthesis to some extent, but the **liver** is the only tissue for the **conversion of excess cholesterol to bile salts**, for excretion from the body in the bile.

Since high levels of cholesterol in the blood have been linked with atherosclerosis, the statin group of drugs has been designed to reduce cholesterol synthesis by inhibiting the HMG CoA reductase enzyme. Cholesterol can be synthesized from acetyl CoA but the pathway is irreversible, and cholesterol cannot be used as a source of energy.

Cholesterol consists of four fused rings and an eight-membered hydrocarbon chain. It is synthesized from acetyl CoA. The first two reactions of the pathway are similar to that of ketogenesis, with the formation of HMG CoA. The **rate limiting step** is the synthesis of mevalonic acid, catalysed by HMG CoA reductase. It requires the reducing properties of 2NADPH and releases acetyl CoA. A five-carbon isoprene unit is then formed from mevalonic acid using ATP. A series of condensation reactions between isoprene units follows, which ends in the formation of squalene, a 30-carbon compound. Squalene is converted to lanosterol by hydroxylation then cyclization. The conversion of lanosterol to cholesterol is a multi-step process that involves many enzymes located in the endoplasmic reticulum. Thus, cholesterol synthesis occurs in the endoplasmic reticulum and the cytoplasm of all cells in the body.

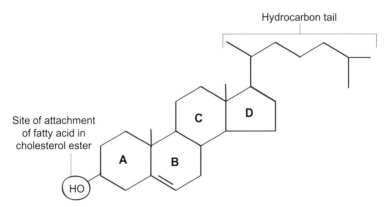

HMG CoA reductase is an intrinsic membrane protein of the endoplasmic reticulum. It is the rate limiting enzyme in the **cholesterol synthesis pathway**. **Glucagon** inhibits HMG CoA reductase whereas **insulin** favours the formation of the active form of the enzyme. This enzyme also experiences **feedback inhibition** by its end product – **cholesterol**.

Answers
18. T T F T F
19. T F F T T
20. T T F T F

21. Regarding lipoprotein particles

a. Chylomicrons carry the least triacylglycerol
b. High density lipoprotein contains the highest percentage of protein
c. Liver receptors recognize apoC on chylomicrons
d. Very low density lipoprotein transports endogenously synthesized triacylglycerol
e. Low density lipoprotein carries cholesterol to extrahepatic tissues

22. True or false? LDL receptors

a. On cell surface membranes recognize the apoB100 present in LDL
b. Are defective in familial hypercholesterolaemia
c. Are downregulated if cholesterol in the circulation is high
d. Are located in clathrin-lined pits in the target cell membrane
e. Are found with different specificity towards oxidized LDL on macrophage cell membranes

23. Regarding chylomicrons

a. Carry dietary triacylglycerol
b. Are assembled in the mitochondria of gut epithelial cells
c. Are the only lipoproteins with apoB48
d. Contain the enzyme lipoprotein lipase
e. Remnants are removed from the circulation by the liver

24. Functions of HDL include

a. Transfer of apoC to very low density lipoprotein to activate lipoprotein lipase
b. Esterification of free cholesterol by the LCAT enzyme
c. Transfer of cholesterol esters to the liver for excretion
d. Transport of fat soluble vitamins from the intestine to the liver
e. Degrade triacylglycerol

25. HDL levels in the blood increase with

a. A high fat diet
b. Regular exercise
c. Smoking
d. Moderate alcohol intake
e. The use of statins

HDL, high density lipoprotein; LDL, low density lipoprotein; VLDL, very low density lipoprotein; IDL, intermediate density lipoprotein; TAG, triacylglycerol; FA, fatty acid; LCAT, lecithin:cholesterol acyltransferase; apo, apoprotein

EXPLANATION: LIPID TRANSPORT

Lipoprotein particles **transport** lipids in the blood to the appropriate tissues. The core is **neutral lipid** (TAG and cholesterol esters) and is surrounded by a shell of **apoproteins**, **cholesterol** and **phospholipid**. Chylomicrons have the lowest density and carry the most lipid. **HDLs** have the greatest density and carry the most protein.

The liver assembles **VLDLs** from endogenously synthesized TAG. They are secreted into the bloodstream where they are degraded by lipoprotein lipase sitting in the walls of capillaries of the adipose tissue, and near the heart and muscle. TAG is removed and broken down to FAs and glycerol, which are taken up by peripheral tissues or donated to HDL. VLDL then becomes IDL, which loses all apoproteins to HDL to form **LDL**.

LDL is the main cholesterol carrier to any tissue that is not the liver. It delivers cholesterol to the interior of a cell through recognition of apoB100 by LDL receptors. LDL receptors cluster in pits lined with clathrin in the plasma membrane. A **deficiency** in LDL receptors (such as is found in individuals with familial hypercholesterolaemia) is an important factor in the development of **atherosclerosis**, since it results in high levels of cholesterol accumulating in the plasma.

Chylomicrons are assembled from **TAG** in the intestine. Their apoprotein components are synthesized and modified in the rough endoplasmic reticulum but the chylomicron itself is assembled in the Golgi. Chylomicrons are synthesized with a unique apoB48 on their surface, but also acquire apoE and apoCII once they are in the circulation. The apoCII allows the chylomicrons to interact with lipoprotein in the capillaries of the adipose tissue to release most of the triglyceride. Lipoprotein lipase hydrolyses chylomicron TAG to monoacylglycerol, FA and glycerol so that they can enter the adipocyte where TAG is re-synthesized and stored. Chylomicron remnants containing cholesterol and fat soluble vitamins are removed from the circulation by the liver.

HDL is **synthesized** in the liver and released to the bloodstream by exocytosis. It acts as a **reservoir** of **apolipoproteins** for the metabolism of other plasma lipoproteins. It is also able to take back these proteins before other lipoproteins (LDL and chylomicrons) are taken up into peripheral cells or the liver.

HDL also takes up free cholesterol from **extrahepatic** tissues and esterifies it using LCAT, an enzyme that is activated by the apoA-1 component of HDL. Cholesterol esters are then transferred to VLDL and LDL in **exchange for TAG**, or they are transported to the liver, where cholesterol is **converted to bile acids or excreted**.

A high level of HDL in the blood is associated with a lower risk of atherosclerosis. HDL levels are generally lower in women than in men. Factors that seem to increase HDL levels in the blood, and thus give protection against atherosclerosis, are regular aerobic exercise and moderate alcohol intake. Factors that are associated with low HDL levels are smoking and a high fat diet (especially high in saturated fats). Statin drugs have been shown to be very effective in lowering circulating LDL levels, but have not been shown to alter HDL levels significantly.

Answers

21. F T F T T
22. T T T T T
23. T F T F T
24. T T T F F
25. F T F T F

26. Fill in the gaps in the following table

Name	Source(s)	Destination	Apoprotein component	Main lipid component
HDL	Liver	Liver	ApoA ApoE ApoC	...1... ...1...
LDL	Liver	...2...	ApoB100	Cholesterol
VLDL	Liver	Peripheral tissue	...3...	TAG
Chylomicrons	...4...	Peripheral tissue	ApoB48 ApoC ApoE	Mostly TAG

HDL, high density lipoprotein; LDL, low density lipoprotein; VLDL, very low density lipoprotein; TAG, triacylglycerol; FA, fatty acid; IDL, intermediate density lipoprotein; TCA, tricarboxylic acid; CM, chylomicron; DHAP, dihydroxyacetone phosphate; TAG, triacylglycerol; FA, fatty acid; ApoB, apoprotein B; ApoC, apoprotein C; LP lipase, lipoprotein lipase; ApoE, apoprotein E

EXPLANATION: PLASMA LIPOPROTEINS

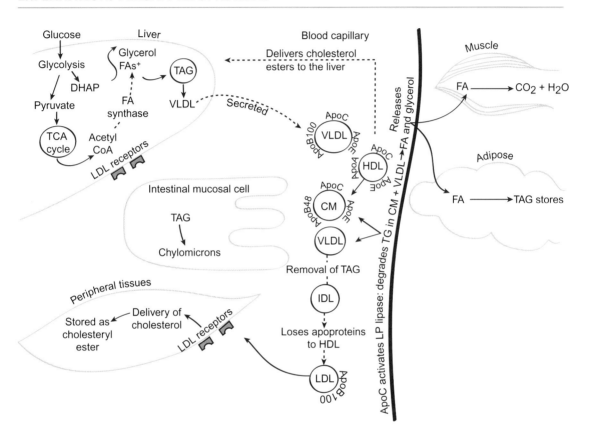

Answers

26. 1 – Cholesterol; 2 – Peripheral tissue and liver; 3 – ApoB100, apoC, apoE; 4 – Small intestine

27. Ketogenesis

a. Only takes place in the liver
b. Forms acetone as a side product
c. Occurs continuously at a low level in the body
d. Is stimulated by a high fat diet
e. Depends on the ratio of NADH to NAD

28. Regarding the utilization of ketone bodies

a. It takes place in the liver
b. It takes place in the kidney
c. It requires the enzyme thiophorase
d. Acetone is useful as a fuel to the brain
e. Ketone bodies require carriers across the blood–brain barrier

29. Regulation of ketone metabolism

a. List three conditions where ketone body synthesis is increased
b. Name three tissues where ketone bodies are metabolized

30. Ketonaemia and ketonuria

a. Occurs when the rate of ketone body formation exceeds the rate of their use
b. Is seen in untreated diabetes mellitus type 1
c. Causes a severe alkalosis
d. Can be detected by characteristic sweet smelling breath
e. Causes dehydration

31. Ketone bodies

a. Are formed within 12 hours of fasting
b. Continue to rise in the plasma with prolonged starvation
c. Stimulate an increase in insulin secretion by the pancreas
d. Can cause a respiratory alkalosis
e. Are utilized by the brain to spare glucose

NAD, nicotinamide adenine dinucleotide; NADH, reduced form of nicotinamide adenine dinucleotide; TCA, tricarboxylic acid; KB, ketone body; FA, fatty acid; HMG CoA, 3-hydroxy-3-methylglutaryl CoA; NAD$^+$, oxidized form of nicotinamide adenine dinucleotide; 3HBD, 3-hydroxbutyrate dehydrogenase

EXPLANATION: KETONE BODY SYNTHESIS

Ketogenesis (KB synthesis) takes place when **acetyl CoA production exceeds the oxidative capacity of the liver**. The acetyl CoA is derived from **FA**. KBs can then be transported to other tissues where they are reconverted back to acetyl CoA and **oxidized** in the **TCA cycle**.

KBs are necessary to provide energy to the tissues during starvation. Although the liver actively produces KBs, it cannot oxidize them because it lacks **thiophorase**. **Extrahepatic tissues** with mitochondria can utilize KBs, including the **brain**. Acetone is a non-metabolizable side-product of ketogenesis. The pathway of ketone metabolism is shown below.

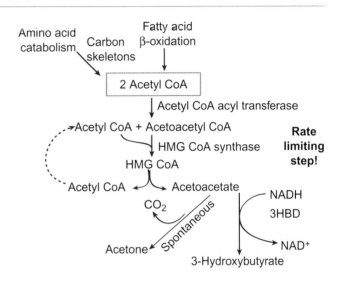

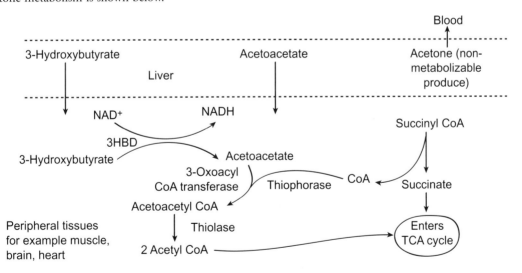

High concentration of KBs in the blood (**ketonaemia**) eventually result in a high level of KBs in the urine (**ketonuria**). Ketonaemia can cause **acidosis** as each KB loses a proton as it circulates in the body, lowering the pH of the blood. Excretion of KBs in the urine causes an osmotic diuresis, leading to dehydration. **This is seen in conditions of starvation, diabetes mellitus and when a high fat, low carbohydrate diet is consumed (29a)**.

Answers
27. T T T T T
28. F T T F F
29. See explanation
30. T T F T T
31. F T T F T

32. Regarding protein metabolism

a. The amino acid pool contains 100 g amino acids
b. Protein turnover is 300–400 g/day
c. Collagen has a half-life of just days
d. The primary role of dietary protein is as a fuel
e. Proteins rich in sequences containing proline, glutamate, serine and threonine are rapidly degraded

33. Indicate whether the following proteins are turned over in (A) hours, (B) days, (C) weeks

1. Albumin
2. Haemoglobin
3. Collagen
4. Insulin
5. Glucagon

34. True or false? Aminotransferases

a. Catalyse irreversibly the transfer of an α-amino group to α-ketoglutarate
b. Contain a prosthetic group derived from vitamin B12
c. Are only present in the mitochondria of cells
d. Act on all amino acids
e. Can be used to monitor for tissue damage

ALT, alanine aminotransferase; AST, aspartate aminotransferase

EXPLANATION: PROTEIN TURNOVER

The **breakdown of amino acids** plays an important part in whole body **nitrogen metabolism**. The amino acid pool consists of **free amino acids** (approximately 100 g) released by hydrolysis of dietary or tissue protein. It is a result of proteins being continuously synthesized and degraded (protein turnover). Average human protein turnover is 300–400 g/day. Structural proteins tend to have a longer half-life than more highly regulated proteins such as hormones. Certain amino acid sequences in the N terminal region of proteins (for example proline, glutamate, serine, threonine) are associated with rapid turnover rates.

Transamination involves the funnelling of amino groups from amino acids to form glutamate. It is the first step in the breakdown of amino acids. Glutamate may be:

• Oxidatively deaminated
• Used for the synthesis of non-essential amino acids

Aminotransferases catalyse the reaction reversibly using a prosthetic group, pyridoxal phosphate, derived from **vitamin B6**. Transamination reactions result in the formation of L-**glutamate** (the new amino acid) and an **α-keto acid**. Lysine and threonine do not take part in transamination reactions.

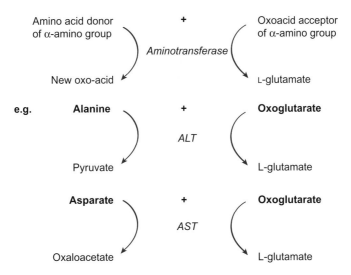

Aminotransferases are intracellular enzymes, present in both cytosolic and mitochondrial locations. Any damage to tissue can be assessed by the leakage of these enzymes from cells, and therefore their presence in the plasma. ALT and AST are particularly useful in assessing liver disease and myocardial infarction.

Answers
32. T T F F T
33. 1 – B, 2 – C, 3 – C, 4 – A, 5 – A
34. F F F F T

35. Oxidative deamination of glutamate

a. May be catalysed by glutamate dehydrogenase
b. Can occur in the kidney
c. Releases ammonia
d. Can only use NAD^+ as a coenzyme
e. Is inhibited by ATP

36. True or false? Ammonia

a. Is highly toxic to the central nervous system
b. Is released from glutamine by glutaminase
c. Is released from glutamate by glutamate dehydrogenase
d. Is formed by bacterial degradation of urea in the intestine
e. Is released on catabolism of purines and pyrimidines

37. Concerning the urea cycle

a. It takes place in the liver hepatocytes
b. Urea production continues during starvation
c. The first two reactions occur in the mitochondria
d. Citrulline is transported into the mitochondria
e. Aspartate provides both nitrogen atoms of urea

38. Carbamoyl phosphate synthetase I

a. Catalyses the rate limiting step of the urea cycle
b. Is activated by citrulline
c. Requires two ATP molecules for each molecule of carbamoyl phosphate made
d. Also participates in pyrimidine synthesis
e. Acts outside the mitochondrial matrix

NAD+, oxidized form of nicotinamide adenine dinucleotide; ATP, adenosine triphosphate; NADH, reduced form of nicotinamide adenine dinucleotide; NADPH, reduced form of nicotinamide adenine dinucleotide phosphate; CNS, central nervous system

EXPLANATION: AMINO ACID METABOLISM

Glutamate deamination is the main route of **nitrogen** removal in the body. Glutamate dehydrogenase is a mitochondrial enzyme in the liver and the kidney. It can use **NADH** or **NADPH** as **coenzymes** for its catalytic activity.

Hyperammonaemia is toxic to the CNS. Sources of ammonia include oxidative **deamination of glutamate**, **glutamine breakdown by glutaminase**, **bacterial action on urea** in the intestine, amines obtained from the **diet**, **purine** and **pyrimidine** catabolism.

Urea is the form in which **amino groups** derived from amino acids are **disposed** of from the body. One nitrogen atom of the urea molecule comes from **free ammonia**, the other from **aspartate**. All but two of the reactions of the cycle occur in the **cytosol** of liver **hepatocytes**; the other two occur in the mitochondria. Urea is transported to the kidney for excretion into the urine. Urea is produced by the liver even during starvation, as skeletal muscle proteins are broken down to release amino acids to act as gluconeogenic precursors. The amino group is removed from these amino acids and converted into urea, which is then excreted in the urine.

Carbamoyl phosphate is formed from CO_2 and NH_3 (or more accurately NH_4^+ as it exists at the pH within the body) in the mitochondrial matrix, catalysed by carbamoyl phosphate synthetase I, **which is the rate limiting step of urea synthesis**. *N*-Acetylglutamate regulates this step – this compound increases intrahepatically following ingestion of a protein-rich meal.

See page 51 for the reactions of the urea cycle and their subcellular locations.

Answers
35. T T T F T
36. T T T T T
37. T T T F F
38. T F T F F

39. Fill in the gaps in the following diagram of the urea cycle, using the list of words below. You may use each word once, more than once, or not at all

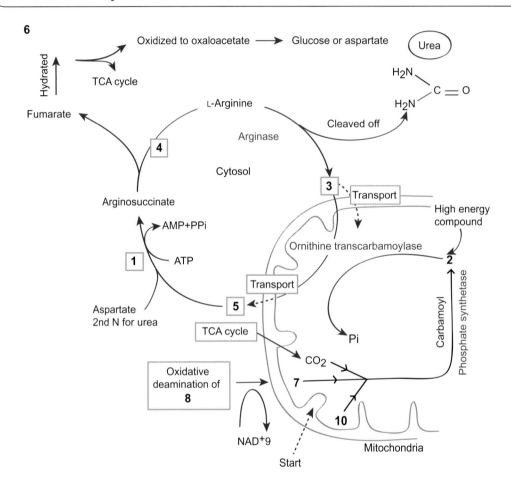

Options

A. Arginosuccinate synthase
C. Malate
F. NADH
H. Ammonia
J. Glutamate

B. ATP
D. L-Ornithine
G. Carbamoyl phosphate
I. L-Citrulline
K. Arginosuccinate lyase

TCA, tricarboxylic acid; AMP, adenosine monophosphate; ATP, adenosine triphosphate; Pi, inorganic phosphate; NADH, reduced form of nicotinamide adenine dinucleotide; PPi, pyrophosphate; NAD^+, oxidized form of nicotinamide adenine dinucleotide

EXPLANATION: UREA CYCLE

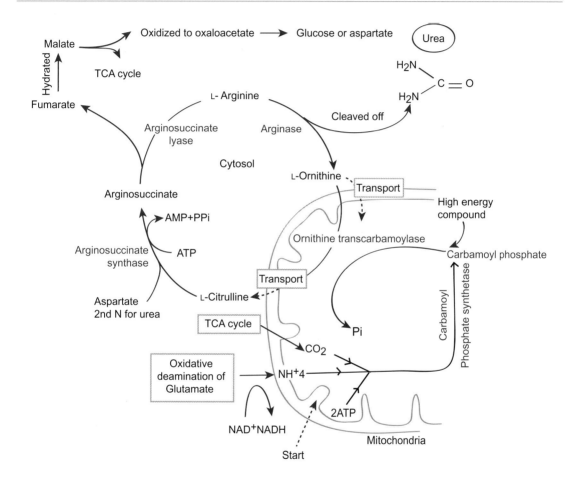

40. True or false? The following amino acids are glucogenic

    a. Alanine
    b. Leucine
    c. Asparagine
    d. Phenylalanine
    e. Tyrosine

41. The following are non-essential amino acids

    a. Tyrosine
    b. Arginine
    c. Threonine
    d. Tryptophan
    e. Cysteine

42. True or false? Phenylketonuria

    a. Is the most common inborn error of amino acid metabolism
    b. Results in elevated plasma levels of phenylalanine
    c. Can be completely reversed by restricting dietary phenylalanine
    d. Causes hyperpigmentation of the eyes and hair
    e. Rarely causes mental retardation

TCA, tricarboxylic acid; PKU, phenylketonuria

EXPLANATION: DIETARY ASPECTS OF AMINO ACIDS

Amino acids may be classified as **glucogenic** or **ketogenic** depending on the nature of their carbon skeletons once their amino groups have been removed. **Leucine** and **lysine** are the only exclusively ketogenic amino acids found in proteins. **Tyrosine** and **phenylalanine** are both glucogenic and ketogenic. Catabolism of glucogenic amino acids yields pyruvate or intermediates of the TCA cycle. Ketogenic amino acids yield acetyl CoA or acetoacetate.

Ten of the 20 amino acids are defined as 'essential', that means that these 10 amino acids need to be taken pre-formed in the diet to maintain good health. The other 10 'non essential' amino acids can be synthesized from commonly available intermediates.

In humans, the dietary essential amino acids are: valine, methionine, histidine, leucine, phenylalanine, lysine, isoleucine, tryptophan, threonine and arginine (arginine and histidine are probably only essential in children and during convalescence).

The list can be remembered easily by the 'memory jogger' rhyme: Very Many Hairy Little Pigs Live In The Torrid Argentine.

PKU is an inherited disorder of amino acid metabolism, with an incidence of 1 in 11000 live births in the UK, and thus is relatively common. It is caused by a deficiency of the enzyme phenylhydroxylase, which is the first step of phenylalanine degradation (and also the route for synthesis of tyrosine, melanin, dopamine, etc). If unrecognized, and untreated, the absence of the enzyme phenylalanine in the blood, which in turn causes damage to the developing brain in babies and young children. Clinical features of untreated PKU inclue mental retardation, seizures, hyperactivity, and hypopigmentation of the eyes and hair.

In the UK, screening of all babies for the PKU condition is carried out within a few days of birth, affected babies are maintained on a diet low in phenylalanine and this continues throughout childhood. The condition is not curable, but the neurological complications can be minimized by careful attention to the prescribed diet.

Answers
40. T F T T T
41. T F F F T
42. T T F F F

SECTION

3

METABOLIC INTEGRATION AND METABOLIC DISORDERS

- GENERAL METABOLISM   56
- BIOMOLECULES AND METABOLIC REACTIONS 58
- ENZYME SUBSTRATES AND ENZYME REACTIONS   60
- ENZYME COFACTORS   62
- OXIDATION/REDUCTION REACTIONS   64
- ENZYME DISORDERS   66
- G6PD DEFICIENCY   68
- FED, FASTING AND STARVATION STATES (i)   70
- FED, FASTING AND STARVATION STATES (ii)   72
- DIABETES   74
- DIABETES TYPES I AND II   76

3

METABOLIC INTEGRATION AND METABOLIC DISORDERS

1. True or false? Examples of catabolic processes include

a. Glycolysis
b. Gluconeogenesis
c. Lipolysis
d. Glycogenesis
e. Lipogenesis

2. True or false? The liver

a. Is the site of the urea cycle
b. Cannot use ketone bodies as an energy source
c. Is the site of purine synthesis
d. Stores most of the body's glycogen
e. Does not synthesize fatty acids

3. Concerning fuel storage, which of the following are true?

a. An average adult stores most glycogen in muscle tissue
b. An average adult has stores of liver glycogen to last about one day
c. Glycogen is stored in extracellular granules
d. By weight, glycogen yields about twice as much energy as fat
e. Glycogen is stored in tissues together with a large amount of 'bound' water molecules

KB, ketone body

EXPLANATION: GENERAL METABOLISM

Catabolic processes involve the breakdown of molecules. The suffix -*lysis* derives from the Greek *lusis* meaning a loosening and indicates a process or decomposition or breaking down. The suffix -*genesis* on the other hand indicates a process of development or generation.

The liver is a major metabolic organ. It is the location of the urea cycle, purine synthesis and is the main site of lipid synthesis. It is also the site of KB synthesis, though it is unable to utilize KBs for energy as it lacks the enzymes 3-ketoacyl CoA transferase or succinyl CoA transferase (also known as thiophorase). Approximately 10 per cent of the liver's mass is glycogen, compared with 1–2 per cent of the mass of muscle. However, as there is far more muscle than liver in the body, about two-thirds of the body's glycogen by weight is stored in muscle.

Fat is a far more efficient way to store energy than glycogen; weight for weight, fat yields about twice as much energy as glycogen. An 'average' 70 kg adult male stores about 100 g of glycogen in his liver, but four times as much in muscle tissue. Glycogen granules are stored intracellularly and occur in most tissues, though most glycogen is found in the liver and muscle cells. Glycogen stores are bulky, as the hydrophilic polymer is associated with a large amount of 'bound' water molecules. This limits the amount of carbohydrate that can be stored in the body as glycogen, and most of the long-term fuel storage is in the form of triglyceride fat in adipose tissue.

Answers

1. T F T F F
2. T T T F F
3. T T F F T

4. Which of the following molecules are depicted in the chemical structures below?

A. Oleic acid
B. Palmitic acid
C. Glucose
D. Sucrose
E. Glycine
F. Glycerol
G. Malonyl CoA
H. Cholesterol
I. Acetyl CoA
J. Acyl CoA

1

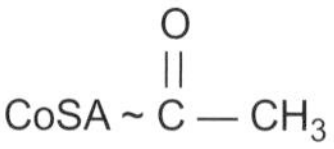

$$CoSA \sim \overset{\overset{\textstyle O}{\|}}{C} - CH_3$$

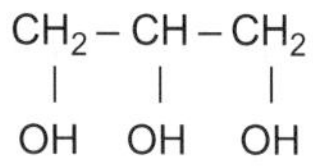

2

$$CH_2 - CH - CH_2$$
$$\;\;|\quad\;\;|\quad\;\;|$$
$$OH \quad OH \quad OH$$

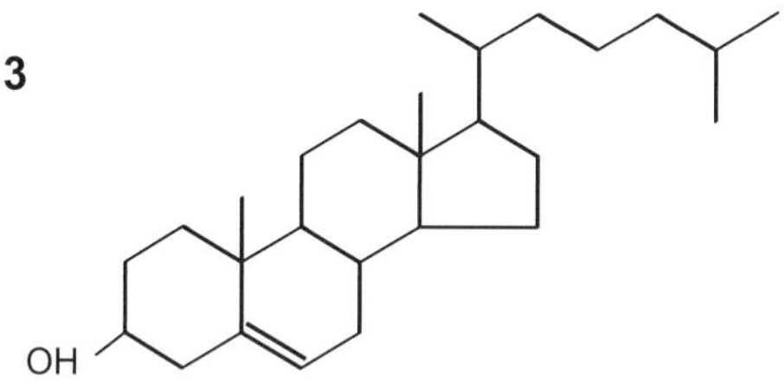

4 $CH_3\,(CH_2)_{14}\,COOH$

3

5

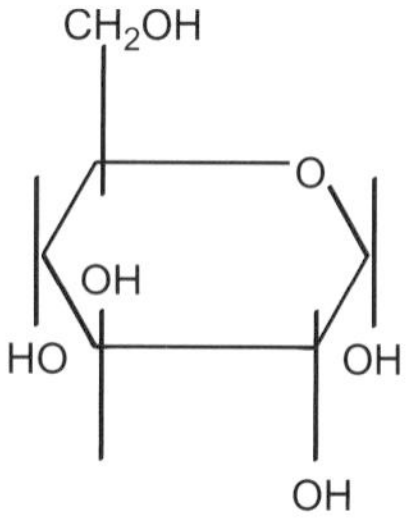

5. Which of the following pairings of metabolic pathways and the locations in which they occur are correct?

a. Glycolysis / mitochondria
b. Fat oxidation / mitochondria
c. Glycogen synthesis / smooth endoplasmic reticulum
d. Citric acid cycle / mitochondria
e. Oxidative phosphorylation / cytosol

6. Which of the pairs of enzyme / reaction type catalysed are correct?

a. Aldolase / isomerism
b. Hexokinase / phosphorylation
c. Aconitase / isomerism
d. Enolase / dehydration
e. Malate dehydrogenase / oxidation-reduction

EXPLANATION: BIOMOLECULES AND METABOLIC REACTIONS

Metabolic pathways that occur in the cytosol include glycolysis, glycogen synthesis and triglyceride synthesis. The processes of fat oxidation, the citric acid cycle and oxidative phosphorylation all take place in the mitochondria.

The reaction in glycolysis catalysed by aldolase is the cleavage of a six-carbon compound into two three-carbon compounds. An isomerism is the conversion of a compound into an isomer of itself, i.e. the substrate and product have the same chemical formula. Hexokinase phosphorylates glucose. Aconitase is an isomerase converting citrate ($C_6H_5O_7$) to isocitrate ($C_6H_5O_7$).

Answers

4. 1 – I, 2 – F, 3 – H, 4 – B, 5 – C
5. F T F T F
6. F T T T T

7. Theme – Enzyme reactions

Match the following enzymes to the descriptions listed below

A. Citrate synthase
C. Phosphofructokinase
E. Malate dehydrogenase
G. Glycerol kinase
I. Pyruvate dehydrogenase

B. Ornithine transcarbamylase
D. Arginase
F. Acetyl CoA carboxylase
H. Hexokinase
J. Lactate dehydrogenase

1. The action of this enzyme on glucose traps it in the cell as the product of the reaction cannot cross the cell membrane
2. The action of this enzyme in anaerobic conditions reduces pyruvate and regenerates NAD^+ in the cytosol
3. This enzyme complex, located on the inner mitochondrial membrane, consists of three enzymes and produces acetyl CoA
4. This enzyme catalyses the conversion of a product of triglyceride hydrolysis to a substrate of the glycolysis pathway
5. This liver enzyme of the urea cycle produces urea and ornithine by cleavage of an amino acid

8. Match the following molecules to the list of reactions involving oxaloacetate below

A. Glucose
C. Glycine
E. Citrate
G. Pyruvate
I. α-Ketoglutarate

B. Malate
D. Succinate
F. Phosphoenolpyruvate
H. Aspartate
J. Glyceraldehyde 3-phosphate

1. NADH is used to reduce oxaloacetate to this compound which is part of a shuttle mechanism for transferring electrons to the electron transport chain
2. Oxaloacetate combines with acetyl CoA to form this compound in the citric acid cycle
3. Transamination of this amino acid forms oxaloacetate
4. Oxaloacetate is a direct precursor of this compound in the gluconeogenesis pathway
5. Oxaloacetate is formed from this compound in the mitochondrial matrix as part of the gluconeogenesis pathway

---

NAD^+, oxidized form of nicotinamide adenine dinucleotide; NADH, reduced form of nicotinamide adenine dinucleotide; FA, fatty acid

EXPLANATION: ENZYME SUBSTRATES AND ENZYME REACTIONS

Hexokinase phosphorylates uncharged glucose to form negatively charged glucose 6-phosphate; as there is no membrane carrier for this compound it is unable to escape the cytosol. In anaerobic conditions the NAD^+ required by glycolysis is regenerated by the conversion of pyruvate to lactate by lactate dehydrogenase. Pyruvate dehydrogenase is a complex of three enzymes that generates acetyl CoA and NADH. Triglyceride hydrolysis produces three FAs and a molecule of glycerol. Glycerol can be converted to glycerol 3-phosphate by the enzyme glycerol kinase. Cleavage of arginine by arginase generates urea and ornithine in the urea cycle.

The irreversible step of glycolysis catalysed by pyruvate kinase is bypassed in gluconeogenesis by conversion of pyruvate first to oxaloacetate, then conversion of oxaloacetate to phosphoenolpyruvate by phosphoenolpyruvate carboxykinase. The transfer of the amino group from glutamate to oxaloacetate produces aspartate, catalysed by the enzyme aspartate aminotransferase. Malate dehydrogenase converts oxaloacetate to malate in the malate–aspartate shuttle.

Oxaloacetate is an intermediate of many metabolic pathways. It also plays a role in the malate–aspartate shuttle, which transfers high energy electrons into mitochondria. Citrate is formed by the condensation of oxaloacetate with acetyl CoA. A transamination reaction transfers an amino group from an amino acid to an α-keto acid. Transfer of the amino group from aspartate to α-ketoglutarate forms oxaloacetate and glutamate. In gluconeogenesis, pyruvate is carboxylated in mitochondria to form oxaloacetate. After transfer to the cytosol, the enzyme phosphoenolpyruvate carboxykinase catalyses the conversion of oxaloacetate to phosphoenolpyruvate.

Answers
7. 1 – H, 2 – J, 3 – I, 4 – G, 5 – D
8. 1 – B, 2 – E, 3 – H, 4 – F, 5 – G

9. The diagram shows the reaction catalysed by the pyruvate dehydrogenase complex. Select labels 1–5 from the following list

Options

A. H_2O
B. CO_2
C. $FAD \rightarrow FADH_2$
D. $NAD^+ \rightarrow NADH + H^+$
E. Acyl CoA
F. Biotin
G. Lactate
H. CoA
I. Acetyl CoA
J. Thiamine pyrophosphate

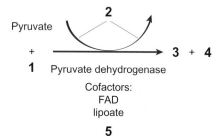

Pyruvate

2

+

1   Pyruvate dehydrogenase   3 + 4

Cofactors:
FAD
lipoate

5

10. True or false? The malate-aspartate shuttle

a. Transports NADH electrons into the mitochondrial matrix
b. Regenerates NAD^+ in the cytosol
c. Is located mainly in cardiac muscle and liver cells
d. Involves reduction of oxaloacetate to malate in the cytosol
e. Involves conversion of oxaloacetate to aspartate in the cytosol

11. With respect to the structure and metabolism of purines

a. Purines have a triple ring structure
b. Nucleosides consist of a purine attached to a pentose sugar
c. Most purines in the body derive from dietary intake
d. Purine synthesis takes place in all cells
e. Breakdown of purines in humans produces uric acid

12. The pentose phosphate pathway

a. Produces NADPH
b. Takes place in the mitochondrial matrix
c. Produces CO_2
d. Is important in the synthesis of nucleotides
e. Can only take place in aerobic conditions

FADH₂, reduced form of flavine adenine dinucleotide; FAD, flavine adenine dinucleotide; NAD⁺, oxidized form of nicotinamide adenine dinucleotide; NADH, reduced form of nicotinamide adenine dinucleotide; NADPH, reduced form of nicotinamide adenine dinucleotide phosphate; NADP, nicotinamide adenine dinucleotide phosphate

EXPLANATION: ENZYME COFACTORS

The pyruvate dehydrogenase complex consists of three enzymes that catalyse the irreversible production of acetyl CoA from pyruvate and CoA. In aerobic conditions the NADH formed by the reaction can be oxidized in the electron transport chain. Thiamine pyrophosphate is a derivative of thiamin (vitamin B1). Deficiency of vitamin B1 leads to a build up of pyruvate. The extra pyruvate is converted to lactate, creating an acidosis.

The malate–aspartate shuttle is the mechanism by which electrons from NADH produced in the cytosol are transported into mitochondria, as the inner membrane is impermeable to NADH itself. Oxaloacetate is reduced to malate in the cytosol by malate dehydrogenase, in the process oxidizing NADH to replenish cytosolic NAD⁺. The malate–aspartate shuttle is found mainly in cardiac muscle and liver cells, while the glycerol 3-phosphate shuttle operates mainly in brain and skeletal muscle cells. Once malate has entered the mitochondria it is oxidized to oxaloacetate, generating NADH within the mitochondrial matrix. Oxaloacetate is then converted to aspartate, which is transported out of the mitochondria in exchange for glutamate.

Purines have a double ring structure with carbon and nitrogen atoms forming a six-molecule ring attached to a five-molecule ring. Nucleosides are formed by the attachment of a five-carbon sugar to a purine. Purines do not come from the diet – they are either synthesized in the liver or recovered from nucleic acids. Purine synthesis only occurs in the cytosol of liver cells. The breakdown of purines forms uric acid.

The oxidative component of the pentose phosphate pathway produces ribulose 5-phosphate, CO_2 and two molecules of NADH from each molecule of glucose 6-phosphate entering the pathway. The reactions take place in the cytosol. The pathway is important in producing the five-carbon sugars used in nucleotide synthesis. The reactions can take place in anaerobic conditions.

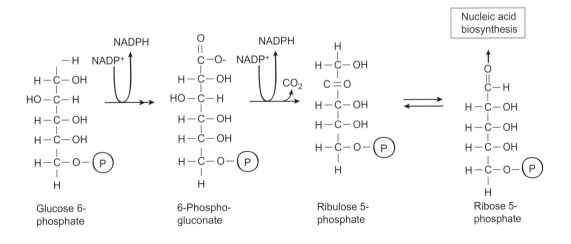

Glucose 6-phosphate   6-Phospho-gluconate   Ribulose 5-phosphate   Ribose 5-phosphate

Answers
9. 1 – H, 2 – D, 3 – I, 4 – B, 5 – J
10. T T T T F
11. F T F F T
12. T F T T F

13. Regarding NADPH (true or false?)

a. NADPH is oxidized by the electron transport chain
b. Is regenerated by the citric acid cycle
c. Is important in fatty acid synthesis
d. Is important in the production of reduced glutathione
e. Is produced by the pentose phosphate pathway

14. Regarding oxidation/reduction cofactors

a. NAD^+ is the oxidation/reduction cofactor required for the pentose phosphate pathway
b. NADH is required for the reaction involving the conversion of pyruvate to lactate in anaerobic glycolysis
c. $FADH_2$ is produced by the succinate dehydrogenation reaction in the TCA cycle
d. Vitamin C (ascorbic acid) is required as the reducing cofactor during the conversion of proline to hydroxyproline in the biosynthesis of collagen
e. Coenzyme Q_{10} (ubiquinone) shuttles electrons between Complex I and Complex III in the electron transport chain

---

FA, fatty acid; NADH, reduced form of nicotinamide adenine dinucleotide; NADPH, reduced form of nicotinamide adenine dinucleotide phosphate; TCA, tricarboxyl acid; NAD^+, oxidized form of nicotinamide adenine dinucleotide; $FADH_2$, reduced form of flavine adenine dinucleotide; GSH, reduced glutathione; GS-SG, oxidized glutathione; $NADP^+$, oxidized form of nicotinamide adenine dinucleotide phosphate

EXPLANATION: OXIDATION/REDUCTION REACTIONS

NADPH is utilized in FA synthesis. Unlike NADH it is not oxidized in the electron transport chain or regenerated by reactions of the citric acid cycle. NADPH is also involved in the defense against oxidative damage in cells.

Glutathione reduces hydrogen peroxide in a reaction catalysed by glutathione peroxidase. After the reaction, glutathione in its oxidized form is inactive and must be reduced to its active state in a reaction requiring NADPH. The only source of NADPH in erythrocytes is the pentose phosphate pathway, and any abnormalities in the pathway such as glucose 6-phosphate dehydrogenase deficiency leads to increased levels of hydrogen peroxide within the cells.

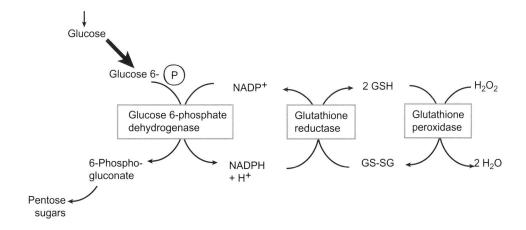

See page 89 for the role of B vitamins and cofactors in metabolism.

Answers
13. F F T T T
14. F T T T T

15. Theme – Disorders of metabolism

Match the following disorders to the descriptions listed below

A. Glucose 6-phosphate dehydrogenase deficiency
B. Acute intermittent porphyria
C. Gout
D. Sickle cell disease
E. Phenylketonuria
F. von Gierke's disease
G. Familial hypercholesterolaemia
H. Type I diabetes
I. Pyruvate kinase deficiency
J. Type II diabetes

1. This condition results from complete loss of the pancreatic beta cells
2. This condition results from impaired insulin secretion and increased insulin resistance
3. This disease results from a lack of one of the enzymes of the pentose phosphate pathway. Sufferers experience haemolysis following exposure to oxidative stressors such as antibiotics and infection
4. This condition results from a lack of glucose 6-phosphatase and causes liver enlargement and fasting hypoglycaemia
5. This condition causes erythrocytes to form prickle shapes and have a reduced lifespan. This causes anaemia, though the oxygen dissociation curve is moved to the right

16. Theme – Disorders of metabolism

Match the following disorders to the descriptions listed below

A. Phenylketonuria
B. Lesch–Nyhan syndrome
C. Glucose 6-phosphate dehydrogenase deficiency
D. Pyruvate kinase deficiency
E. Acute intermittent porphyria
F. Type I diabetes
G. Familial hypercholesterolaemia
H. Type I hyperlipidaemia (lipoprotein lipase or apolipoprotein-C_2 deficiency)
I. Tay-Sachs disease
J. Gout

1. This condition results in inability to remove chylomicrons from the blood. It presents in childhood with eruptive xanthomas, lipaemia retinalis, retinal vein thrombosis, pancreatitis and hepatosplenomegaly
2. This autosomal dominant disorder is usually due to defective low density lipoprotein receptors and can lead to ischaemic heart disease in childhood
3. This autosomal recessive disorder results from a lack of the enzyme that catalyses the conversion of phenylalanine to tyrosine
4. This condition is a rare X-linked disorder of purine metabolism that usually kills in early childhood; it causes kidney stones, arthritis, spasticity and mental retardation
5. This condition is due to an abnormal uric acid metabolism that leads to crystal deposits in joint spaces causing arthritis

---

2,3-BPG, 2,3-bisphosphoglycerate; G6PD, glucose-6-phosphate dehydrogenase; NADPH, reduced form of nicotinamide adenine dinucleotide phosphate; PKU, phenylketonuria

EXPLANATION: ENZYME DISORDERS

Many diseases are caused by faults in metabolic processes, often due to abnormal or absent genes coding for enzymes. **Type I diabetes** results from complete loss of pancreatic beta cells, which may be secondary to autoimmune destruction. Type II diabetes is due to reduced or inadequate secretion of insulin and/or peripheral insulin resistance. G6PD is an enzyme of the pentose phosphate pathway. Erythrocytes use the pentose phosphate pathway to generate NADPH which is necessary for deactivation of hydrogen peroxide. **Deficiency of G6PD** leads to increased hydrogen peroxide levels, oxidative damage to and ultimately loss of erythrocytes. Deficiency of glucose 6-phosphatase causes the glycogen storage disorder **von Gierke's disease**. **Pyruvate kinase** deficiency in erythrocytes leads to distortion in their structure and a reduced lifespan. This leads to an anaemia; however, the enzyme deficiency causes a 'backlog' of glycolysis intermediates including 2,3-BPG, which shifts the oxygen desaturation curve to the right.

The classification of hyperlipidaemias is confusing as there are two means of classification – the **Fredrickson** based on the pattern of plasma lipoproteins in each condition, and the **Goldstein** based on the underlying enzyme defects. **Type I hyperlipidaemia (Fredrickson)** is a lipoprotein lipase or apolipoprotein-C2 deficiency. It leads to massive lipid deposition and presents in childhood. **Type IIa hyperlipidaemia (familial hypercholesterolaemia)** is a severe illness, not to be confused with common hypercholesterolaemia. Familial hypercholesterolaemia presents in childhood with deposits of cholesterol in the skin and ischaemic heart disease in adolescence.

PKU is caused by deficiency of phenylalanine hydroxylase that converts phenylalanine to tyrosine. Routine screening for phenylketonuria is undertaken in neonates.

Gout is caused by a disorder of uric acid metabolism that leads to crystal deposition in joint spaces and arthritis.

Lesch–Nyhan syndrome is a rare X-linked disorder of purine metabolism that usually kills in early childhood; it causes kidney stones, arthritis, spacticity and mental retardation.

Answers
15. 1 – H, 2 – J, 3 – A, 4 – F, 5 – I
16. 1 – H, 2 – G, 3 – A, 4 – B, 5 – J

17. Case study

A 20-year-old male Nigerian student presents at A&E with a one-week history of a flu-like illness. Over this period he has become weak and now feels short of breath at rest. On examination he is pale, and his sclera appear to be tinged slightly yellow. Blood tests show that he is anaemic with a haemoglobin of 8.0 g/dL (normal range: 11.5–16 g/dL). His serum bilirubin is found to be raised, and the blood report states that Heinz bodies are seen on the blood film. Some weeks later, enzyme assays confirm the diagnosis.

   a. What is the most likely enzyme deficiency?
   b. Why is the bilirubin level raised?
   c. What is causing the breakdown of red cells? How does this relate to the enzyme deficiency?

18. True or false? Glucose 6-phosphate dehydrogenase (G6PD) deficiency

   a. Is an autosomal recessive disorder
   b. Is more common in Africa than in the UK
   c. Carrier status confers some protection against *Plasmodium falciparum* infection (malaria)
   d. Haemolytic crisis may be induced by certain antibiotics
   e. Haemolytic crisis may be induced by eating broad beans (fava beans)

G6PD, glucose 6-phosphate dehydrogenase; NADPH, reduced form of nicotinamide adenine dinucleotide phosphate; RBC, red blood cell

EXPLANATION: G6PD DEFICIENCY

G6PD is an enzyme of the pentose phosphate pathway. In red cells, decreased G6PD leads to decreased NADPH formation. NADPH activates glutathione, which in turn reduces reactive oxygen intermediates which would otherwise cause cell damage.

G6PD deficiency **(17a)** is the most common erythrocyte enzyme disorder in the world, affecting more than 100 million people worldwide. This genetic condition is very common in the populations of East and Central Africa, the areas round the Mediterranean, the Middle East and South East Asia. The condition is inherited in an X-linked manner, and female carriers have some protection against infection by malaria.

Individuals with this condition have good health until a haemolytic crisis is precipitated by oxidative stress, such as bacterial infections, antibiotics, antimalarial drugs, certain dyes, or the ingestion of fava beans (similar to broad beans). A blood film from a patient who has this condition will often show the presence of Heinz bodies inside the RBCs, which result from the precipitation of oxidized, denatured haemoglobin.

Patients who have had a haemolytic crisis will have raised plasma bilirubin levels because the processes within the liver that are responsible for disposing of bilirubin (formed by the breakdown of haemoglobin) have a limited capacity, and when they reach their limit bilirubin levels rise in the blood. It is bilirubin that causes jaundice – the yellow colouring of skin and sclera. A finding of jaundice is characteristic of haemolysis, in which a sudden breakdown of erythrocytes overloads the haemoglobin degradation and disposal mechanism **(17b)**.

In G6PD deficiency the red cells are destroyed because of a build up of hydrogen peroxide. Hydrogen peroxide is reduced to H_2O by the antioxidant glutathione. The oxidized glutathione produced by this reaction is inactive and is reactivated in a reaction that uses NADPH as a reducing agent. Effective reduction of hydrogen peroxide and other reactive oxygen intermediates therefore requires a continuous supply of NADPH. In erythrocytes, the only source of NADPH is the pentose phosphate pathway, but lack of G6PD inhibits this pathway and hence leads to a build up of reactive oxygen intermediates that oxidize haemoglobin and cell membrane components. This oxidative damage ultimately leads to breakdown of erythrocytes **(17c)**.

Answers

17. See explanation
18. F T T T T

19. Two to four hours after a high carbohydrate meal

a. The liver is engaged in gluconeogenesis
b. Phosphofructokinase is activated
c. Fatty acid synthesis is decreased
d. The brain uses glucose exclusively as fuel
e. Increased levels of insulin inactivate lipoprotein lipase

20. During an overnight fast the liver

a. Increases gluconeogenesis
b. Has enhanced activity of the hexose monophosphate pathway
c. Increases fatty acid oxidation
d. Does not degrade glycogen
e. Increases uptake of branched chain amino acids

21. During starvation

a. Hormone-sensitive lipase is activated by glucagon
b. Not all glycogen in depleted
c. Tissues oxidize fatty acids alone
d. Ketone bodies plateau in the plasma
e. Death is usually a result of infection

TCA, tricarboxylic acid; TAG, triacylglycerol; FA, fatty acid; KB, ketone body

EXPLANATION: FED, FASTING AND STARVATION STATES (i)

Metabolism is principally controlled by the **action of catecholamines, and insulin and glucagon**. They determine whether the body is predominantly in a state of **anabolism** or **catabolism** in response to the availability of nutrients.

THE FED STATE **Two to four hours** after a meal, the body is in the **absorptive** (fed) state. This is a period of anabolism, where there is a **high insulin:glucagon ratio** in the circulation. In the liver, glycolysis is increased, and glycogen synthesis is favoured. There is no gluconeogenesis. Surplus amino acids are used for protein synthesis or deaminated in the liver to pyruvate, acetyl CoA or oxaloacetate, which enter the TCA cycle. FA synthesis is favoured since excess acetyl CoA is converted to malonyl CoA (by acetyl CoA carboxylase). Malonyl CoA inhibits the **carnitine shuttle** which transports FAs to be oxidized in the mitochondria, therefore they have to be stored as TAG in the periphery.

Lipoprotein lipase is activated by high levels of insulin. It acts to extract FAs and glycerol from chylomicrons in the circulation, which are taken up by the adipocytes and re-esterified into TAG to be stored. Insulin inactivates **hormone-sensitive lipase** to ensure that TAG is not degraded. (Be careful not to get the two enzymes confused.) In the fed state the brain and erythrocytes exclusively use glucose as their fuel supply. Muscle uses glucose as its main fuel, and is also able to metabolize branched amino acids (leucine, isoleucine and valine) as well.

THE OVERNIGHT FAST If no food is taken for **a period between 4–12 hours** the body enters the postabsorptive state. The **ratio of insulin to glucagon** is low, and this is therefore a period of catabolism where the body's efforts are focused on **maintaining blood glucose** within the normal range and therefore an adequate fuel supply to the vital organs. The liver **degrades glycogen** to release glucose to the bloodstream, however this store is quickly depleted. **Gluconeogenesis** is therefore increased, using **lactate** (from anaerobic glycolysis), carbon skeletons of amino acids (from protein degradation in the muscle) and glycerol (from hydrolysis of TAG). **Hormone-sensitive lipase** catalyses the breakdown (hydrolysis) of TAG, and is activated by **glucagon**.

FAs from the breakdown of TAG cannot be used for gluconeogenesis, rather they are oxidized in tissues to produce acetyl CoA. **Acetyl CoA inhibits the conversion of pyruvate** (from glycolysis) to acetyl CoA. Therefore **glucose is spared**, and FAs are used as a metabolic fuel instead. The surplus acetyl CoA may exceed the capacity of the TCA cycle, and therefore is converted to KBs. KBs are metabolized by most tissues except erythrocytes, which can only use glucose.

Answers
19. F T F T F
20. T F T F F
21. T F F F T

22. In a normal adult after 24 hours without food

    a. Cortisol release induces muscle protein breakdown
    b. Ketone bodies are formed in the liver
    c. Amino acids and glycerol are used for gluconeogenesis
    d. Urea excretion in urine falls to zero
    e. Liver glycogen is the main source of energy for the brain

23. Complete the passage below by selecting from the list A–J

    A. Acetoacetate
    B. Mitochondria
    C. Acetate
    D. Cytosol
    E. Adipose
    F. Enoyl CoA hydratase
    G. Liver
    H. Succinyl CoA transferase
    I. Three
    J. Two

Ketone bodies are formed from acetyl CoA. The process involves .... molecules of acetyl CoA being combined to form HMG CoA, which then splits to form ....$_2$. Ketone bodies are formed in the ....$_3$ of ....$_4$ cells, but are utilized mainly by cardiac muscle, skeletal muscle and brain cells. Cells that lack the enzyme ....$_5$, such as liver cells, are unable to use ketone bodies as an energy source as this enzyme catalyses a key step in regenerating acetyl CoA from ketone bodies.

24. True or false? Ketogenesis

    a. Occurs in the cytosol of liver cells
    b. Increases in starvation
    c. Increases in uncontrolled type I diabetes
    d. May result in the production of acetone
    e. Results in the production of glucose

HMG CoA, 3-hydroxy-3-methylglutaryl CoA; FA, fatty acid; KB, ketone body; TAG, triacylglycerol

EXPLANATION: FED, FASTING AND STARVATION STATES (ii)

STARVATION   If fasting continues, **muscle protein** is in danger of being depleted because it is being broken down for gluconeogenic substrates. The body develops mechanisms to prevent this happening. Firstly the kidney **reabsorbs** more **KBs** from the filtrate, so that they can be used as fuel for the brain instead of glucose. Secondly muscle oxidizes FAs in preference to KBs. This results in a decreased requirement for gluconeogenesis. The **rising KB concentration** in the plasma causes an **increase in insulin secretion**. Insulin prevents protein breakdown in the muscle, and inhibits TAG hydrolysis in the adipose tissue.

In the early stage of starvation, noradrenaline and cortisol induce breakdown of protein. Generation of KBs from FAs takes place in the liver, while glycerol and amino acids are used for gluconeogenesis. In starvation, uric acid excretion falls by about 50 per cent. Liver glycogen is exhausted after 12–24 hours without food.

KBs are generated from acetyl CoA in liver cell mitochondria. The three KBs are acetoacetate, acetone and 3-hydroxybutyrate. They are carried in the blood to tissues that can use them as an energy source. Liver cells are unable to utilize KBs as fuel, as liver cells lack the enzyme 3-ketoacyl CoA transferase that is necessary to regenerate acetyl CoA from the KBs.

Production of KBs begins in the first few days of starvation and in uncontrolled type I diabetes, in which excessive production can lead to acidosis. Acetone, one of the KBs, has a distinctive smell (like nail varnish remover) and can be detected on the breath. KBs are an alternative source of energy to glucose, KBs do not enter the gluconeogenesis pathway.

Answers
22. T T T F F
23. 1 – I, 2 – A, 3 – B, 4 – G, 5 – H
24. F T T T F

25. With regard to diabetes mellitus

a. Hyperglycaemia is a hallmark of the disease
b. Metabolic changes are similar to those seen in starvation
c. Symptoms arise from the unopposed action of glucagon
d. Lipolysis is reduced
e. Ketoacidosis occurs as a result of protein catabolism

26. The following are features of untreated type I diabetes mellitus

a. Weight gain
b. Excessive thirst
c. Frequent urination
d. Oedema
e. Anaemia

27. In an uncontrolled state type I diabetes mellitus leads to

a. Hyperglycaemia
b. Hypoglycaemia
c. Depletion of liver glycogen stores
d. Increased hepatic ketone synthesis
e. A rise in blood pH

28. Type II diabetes mellitus

a. Leads to low blood glucose concentrations
b. May result from lowered sensitivity of target tissues to insulin
c. Commonly leads to ketoacidosis
d. Is usually caused by autoimmune destruction of pancreatic beta cells
e. May not require insulin therapy

29. With regard to type I and type II diabetes

a. The onset of type I diabetes typically occurs after the age of 60
b. Type II diabetes is caused by autoimmune destruction of pancreatic beta cells
c. Ketoacidosis occurs more frequently in type II diabetes
d. Type II diabetes may require control by insulin
e. Both insulin and non-insulin therapies may cause hypoglycaemia

TAG, triacylglycerol; FA, fatty acid; KB, ketone body; TCA, tricarboxylic acid

EXPLANATION: DIABETES

Diabetes affects 2 per cent of people in the UK. It is thought that its prevalence in the world is set to double in the next 10 years. **Diabetes** may be separated into two groups: **insulin dependent** (type I) and **non-insulin dependent** (type II). **Type I diabetes** is defined as a state of **hyperglycaemia** resulting from a **lack of insulin secretion by the beta cells in the islets of Langerhans of the pancreas**. It is an endocrine autoimmune disease: T cells attack and destroy healthy beta cells. Glucose is available in the bloodstream but the peripheral tissues are **unable to take it up and use it as metabolic fuel**. For this reason the condition is known as 'starvation in the midst of plenty'. **Hyperglycaemia** results in **glucose** in the urine (**glycosuria**), **polyuria**, **weight loss** and **intense thirst** (**polydipsia**). Patients may present with a severe metabolic disturbance known as ketoacidosis.

Type II diabetes is characterized by **insulin deficiency** combined with an **increased resistance** to insulin by the peripheral tissues. It appears to be a disease of ageing. As we get older, beta cells become less efficient and sensitivity to insulin decreases. Many genetic and environmental factors affect the incidence of type II diabetes, for example nutrition, birthweight, obesity and physical activity.

Hyperglycaemia is less marked than in type I diabetes, because there is some insulin function. **Type II diabetics do not become ketoacidotic**. Patients are usually overweight and have slower progressing symptoms. They may present with complications of poorly controlled blood glucose, either **macrovascular** or **microvascular**. Macrovascular complications include **ischaemic heart disease**, **cerebrovascular disease** or **peripheral vascular disease**. Microvascular complications include **retinopathy** (eyes), **nephropathy** (kidney) or **neuropathy** (nerves). Type II diabetes is generally treated through a controlled diet and weight loss.

Diabetics can experience episodes of **hyperglycaemia** after **infection** or **illness** because they do not take their insulin. The boy in the case study (p.77) is hyperglycaemic because he has an insulin deficiency. Therefore peripheral tissues are unable to take up glucose from the blood. The lack of insulin removes inhibition of the alpha cells in the islets of Langerhans so that they secrete an **excess of glucagon**, which has a catabolic effect breaking down glycogen to glucose and **increasing gluconeogenesis**, allowing glucose in the blood to rise further **(31b)**. The stress of the insulin deficiency additionally stimulates catecholamine secretion which has further catabolic effects.

As in the fasted state, during insulin deficiency lipolysis is uninhibited. FAs are released from **adipose tissue** by the hydrolysis of TAG. FAs provide a **fuel** for **muscle** and provide glycerol for gluconeogenesis. However, the production of **acetyl CoA** from FA oxidation in the mitochondria exceeds the capacity of the TCA cycle in the liver. Therefore some of the acetyl CoA is channelled into **KB** formation, which can be used as fuel by many tissues including the brain. In diabetes, since there is no insulin, ketones can rise to a very high level, causing ketoacidosis, and therefore ketonuria. Since acetone is non-metabolizable, it is discharged in the urine **(31a)**.

Ketoacidosis results when the levels of KBs in the plasma **exceed** the **buffering capacity** of the bicarbonate ions in the blood. The metabolic acidosis can naturally be compensated for by what is known as Kussmaul breathing **(31c)**. The low plasma pH stimulates the respiratory centre to produce deep breathing to expel CO_2 from the blood, and compensate for the falling HCO_3^- levels. The following equilibrium shifts to the left $H_2O + CO_2 \leftrightarrow H_2CO_3 \leftrightarrow HCO_3^- + H^+$. There is a limit to hyperventilation but no limit to ketogenesis.

Answers

25. T T T F F
26. F T T F F
27. T F T T F
28. F T F F T
29. F F F T T

30. Case study

A 50-year-old man attends his GP complaining of tiredness, constantly needing to urinate and excessive thirst. He weighs 102 kg and is 180 cm tall. He is found to have a fasting blood sugar level of 13 mmol/L. Glucose is detected in his urine.

    a. What is the most likely diagnosis?

    b. The man is commenced on oral drug therapy. Name two classes of drug that may be appropriate here and their modes of action

    c. Some years later, it is found that the drug therapy is failing to control his disease. What further treatment may benefit him? Name two risks associated with this type of treatment

    d. Calculate his body mass index (BMI)

31. Case study

A 16-year-old boy who is a known diabetic goes on holiday to Mallorca with friends after taking his GCSEs. Whilst away his diet and insulin regime become irregular. On his return to England he suffers from a bout of flu. He decides to cut out his insulin as he is not eating. Over the next few days he feels increasingly unwell with stomach ache, increased urination and thirst. His mum brings him into hospital hyperventilating. His blood pH is low, a glucose reagent stick shows he is hyperglycaemic, and a urine sample tests positive for ketone bodies.

    a. Why are there ketone bodies in his urine?

    b. Why is he hyperglycaemic?

    c. How can he compensate for his acidic blood?

KB, ketone body; BMI, body mass index; GP, general practitioner

EXPLANATION: DIABETES TYPES I AND II

A middle-aged man who is overweight, and complains of excessive thirst is most likely to be suffering from diabetes type II (non-insulin dependent diabetes) **(30)**.

This man gives a classic history of fatigue, polyuria (large volumes of urine produced) and polydipsia (needing to drink large volumes). This is more likely to be type II diabetes than type I as the onset of type II is typically in an older age group and is associated with obesity – this man's BMI is 31.5.

The two main classes of drugs used in treating type II diabetes are the biguanides and the sulfonylureas. Metformin is the only biguanide available in the UK, it increases sensitivity of tissues to insulin and inhibits gluconeogenesis in the liver. The sulfonylureas increase pancreatic insulin secretion. Another drug that can be used is Acarbose, which inhibits the enzyme α-glucosidase, preventing the breakdown of complex carbohydrates to simple sugars **(30b)**.

Insulin therapy may be required in the control of type II diabetes. Insulin is given by subcutaneous injection, usually several times a day in an attempt to mimic the normal physiological variation. The most serious risk with insulin therapy is that of hypoglycaemia. Hypoglycaemia develops if insulin is injected and not followed by a meal and is a medical emergency. Fat hypertrophy may occur if insulin is continually injected into the same site. Rotation of the sites of injection is therefore advised **(30c)**.

BMI is equal to the patient's mass in kilograms divided by the square of their height in metres. In this case, BMI = $102 \div 1.8^2 = 31.48$ **(30d)**. Normal BMI range for men is 20–24.

For explanation of ketosis and hyperglycaemia in diabetes type I, see page 75.

Answers

30. See explanation
31. See explanation

4   GENERAL NUTRITION

- NUTRITIONAL MEASUREMENTS 80
- DIETARY FAT 82
- CARBOHYDRATES 84
- DIETARY PROTEIN 86
- WATER-SOLUBLE VITAMINS 88
- FAT-SOLUBLE VITAMINS 90
- IRON 92
- CALCIUM AND ZINC 94

GENERAL NUTRITION

1. Using the diagram below determine whether the following statements are true or false

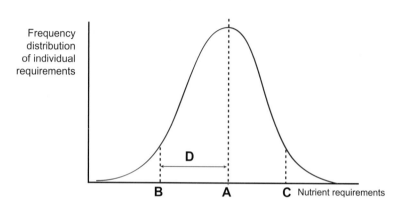

a. **A** represents the estimated average requirement for a group of healthy individuals in a population of a particular nutrient

b. **B** represents the estimated average requirement for a group of healthy individuals in a population of a particular nutrient

c. **C** represents the nutrient values of safe intake

d. **D** is a distance of two standard deviations

e. This graph would be skewed for dietary iron requirements in women

2. Examples of staple foods include

a. Potatoes

b. Rice

c. Milk

d. Bananas

e. Wheat

3. True or false? Daily energy expenditure

a. Is increased in pregnancy

b. Decreases with age

c. Can be measured using a double-labelled H_2O technique

d. Includes the thermic effect of food

e. Is expressed as a multiple of basal metabolic rate

EAR, estimated average requirement; RNI, reference nutrient intake; DRV, dietary reference value; BMR, basal metabolic rate

EXPLANATION: NUTRITIONAL MEASUREMENTS

DRVs have been formulated in the UK by the Committee on Medical Aspects of Food and Nutrition. The requirements for most nutrients in a population are normally distributed. In the graph opposite, **A** is the EAR, the **mean requirement**, for a group of healthy individuals; **B** is the lower RNI – intakes **below** this level are inadequate for most individuals; **C** is the RNI that is a value two standard deviations above the EAR. Intakes at this latter amount meet the needs of 97.5 per cent of the population. For some nutrients there are insufficient data on human requirements to set DRVs; for these nutrients, values of safe intakes are given instead.

The distribution of dietary iron requirements for women is skewed because a minority of women in the population lose 3–4 times more blood than the median value of 30 mL during menstruation.

A staple food is the principal food of a country, usually **cereals or root crops**. In the UK, cereal foods provide 30 per cent of energy, 25 per cent of protein and 50 per cent of total carbohydrate. Although dairy products and high calorie fruits such as bananas and plaintain are valuable food sources, they are not the major source of calories for whole populations of any country.

Daily energy expenditure is the **sum of BMR, thermic effect of food eaten, occupational activities and non-occupational activities**. Energy requirements increase with growth, pregnancy and lactation, (as does expenditure) and decreases with age.

There is no RNI for energy intake since this would depend on the activity of the individual and because adding two standard deviations to the estimated average would give a much larger intake than most people need!

Energy requirements can be measured by the use of doubly labelled water ($^2H_2$ ^{18}O) and following incorporation of the ^2H and the ^{18}O into body fluits and urine. ^2H is incorporated into H_2O, but in contrast, ^{18}O is incorporated into H_2O and CO_2. Labelled H_2O and CO_2 can be measured using indirect mass spectroscopy.

Answers
1. T F F T T
2. T T F F T
3. T T T T F

4. True or false? Dietary fat

a. Is not necessary in the diet
b. Makes food palatable
c. Provides 37 kJ of energy per gram
d. Inhibits the absorption of some vitamins
e. In excess is associated with coronary heart disease

5. Polyunsaturated fatty acids in the diet

a. Can lower serum cholesterol
b. Have no double bonds
c. Are high in the Mediterranean diet
d. Should not be taken with antioxidants
e. Should not exceed 10 per cent of total dietary energy

6. Essential fatty acids

a. Cannot be obtained from the diet
b. Are found in fish oils
c. Cannot be synthesized by the body
d. Contain ω3 and ω6 double bonds
e. Have a *trans* configuration

7. Explain why the 'Mediterranean diet' is thought to be good for the health

FA, fatty acid; LDL, low density lipoprotein

EXPLANATION: DIETARY FAT

Dietary fat is mostly in the form of **triglycerides** – esters of glycerol and free FAs. They are known as unsaturated fats if they have carbon double bonds. A **small amount of fat** is necessary in the diet to provide **polyunsaturated FAs** (also known as **essential FAs**), which cannot be synthesized by the body. Fat has the highest energy yield, and therefore is an important concentrated energy store. It is also necessary for the **absorption of fat soluble vitamins**: A, D, E and K.

Essential fatty acids or polyunsaturated fatty acids **include linoleic acid, α-linolenic acid** (and probably **arachidonic acid** in children). They must be taken in the diet, and are found in fish and vegetable oils. They contain ω3 or ω6 bonds (see page 29).

Cis-unsaturated FAs have a *cis* configuration. They are found in plants and most animal sources. *Trans*-unsaturated fats have a *trans* configuration, and are made artificially by the hydrogenation of long chain FAs, for example when making margarine. There is some concern that *trans* FAs may be associated with atherosclerosis.

Saturated FAs cause an increase in **LDL** and **cholesterol**. Although cholesterol is important as a precursor to **bile formation**, it is also involved in **atheroma formation**. Cholesterol can be lowered by raising the intake of polyunsaturated FAs, however they should be taken with antioxidant nutrients to prevent FA peroxidation.

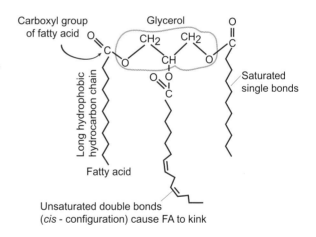

Studies have shown that the incidence of heart disease is lower in Mediterranean countries, such as Greece and Italy, than in northern European countries. It is thought to be because of the difference in diet. The Mediterranean-type diet:

- Is lower in saturated fat
- Contains a higher proportion of fruit and vegetables
- Is higher in monounsaturated fats (oleic acid found in olive oil) **(7)**

Answers

8. True or false? Dietary carbohydrates

a. Have a protein-sparing effect
b. Prevent ketoacidosis
c. Include starch and sucrose
d. Should make up approximately two-thirds of the caloric intake
e. Can be converted to glycogen

9. Dietary fibre

a. Is a non-starch polysaccharide
b. Has a high calorific content
c. Is thought to bind carcinogens
d. Contains cellulose
e. Lowers blood cholesterol

10. High levels of simple sugars such as sucrose in the diet

a. Cause diabetes
b. Are inherently fattening
c. May cause dental caries
d. Cause an increase in blood cholesterol
e. May lead to behavioural abnormalities in children

EXPLANATION: CARBOHYDRATES

Carbohydrates are compounds of **carbon, hydrogen** and **oxygen** in the ratio $C_n:H_{2n}:O_n$. Theoretically they are not essential to the diet, as **amino acids** can be converted to **glucose**. However, carbohydrates allow proteins to be used for growth and maintenance of tissues rather than as fuel, thus they have a protein-sparing effect. Also, they prevent the use of fat as a metabolic fuel, reducing the likelihood of ketoacidosis.

There are three types of carbohydrate: **starch, non-starch polysaccharide and sugars**. Of the simple sugars, disaccharides such as sucrose, maltose and lactose are far more abundant in the diet than monosaccharides such as glucose and fructose. All forms of carbohydrate that can be digested and absorbed can be converted to glycogen for storage in liver or skeletal muscle.

Dietary fibre, also known as **non-starch polysaccharides**, is found in **cereals, vegetables** and **fruit**. It has several beneficial effects on health, including the binding of **carcinogens** to prevent their absorption into the intestine. However, fibre can also bind **trace elements** and **decrease** the absorption of fat soluble vitamins. As non-starch polysaccharides include cellulose, which cannot be digested and absorbed in the human digestive tract, they do not contribute to the calorie intake of the body.

There is no evidence to suggest that sugars have detrimental effects on our health up to a level of intake as much as 30 per cent of our total dietary requirement. However, sucrose is a major cause of **dental caries**. Studies have shown a very strong positive correlation between the incidence of caries and sugar consumption. It is thought that frequency of sugary foods plays a more significant role than actual amount.

Answers
8. T T T T T
9. T F T T T
10. F F T T F

11. Concerning protein and the diet

a. High quality proteins contain all the essential amino acids
b. 'Limiting' amino acids are the essential amino acids present in the lowest concentration in the protein
c. Protein complementation is supplementation of a low protein diet with carbohydrate
d. Adults require three times the protein intake per day of a newborn baby
e. Excessive protein intake is likely to be harmful to the body

12. The following disorders can be caused by dietary deficiency or malnutrition

a. Diabetes mellitus
b. Hypothyroidism
c. Cushing's disease
d. Blindness
e. Osteoporosis

13. Nitrogen balance is positive

a. During pregnancy
b. Following trauma
c. On recovery from an emaciating disease
d. During starvation
e. In children

PEM, protein energy malnutrition

EXPLANATION: DIETARY PROTEIN

The **need for dietary protein** stems from the need for certain amino acids (the **essential amino acids**!) that cannot be synthesized in the body. **High quality** proteins have a high utilization value because they contain **all the essential amino acids**. **Protein complementation** is the mixing of dietary proteins with different limiting amino acids to raise their combined utilization value.

It is important not to confuse **nutritional deficiency** with **endocrinological dysfunction**. Diabetes is caused by insulin deficiency or resistance, resulting in uncontrolled fluctuations in blood glucose. Cushing's disease is caused by glucocorticoid excess. Blindness may be caused by vitamin A deficiency, and **osteomalacia** (not osteoporosis) may be caused by **vitamin D deficiency**. **Hypothyroidism** is usually caused by a defect in thyroid function, but can also be due to a dietary deficiency of iodine.

Nitrogen balance occurs in normal adults when nitrogen intake in the **diet** is **equal** to the nitrogen **excreted** in the urine, faeces and sweat.

A positive balance indicates that nitrogen is being retained by the body and that protein is being laid down. This occurs in growing children, pregnancy and recovery from an emaciating disease.

PEM results from a diet **inadequate** in **protein** and **energy**. It manifests as **growth failure**, **marasmus** or **kwashiorkor**.

14. Regarding water-soluble vitamins

a. Certain vitamins can be synthesized by humans
b. B group vitamins serve as coenzymes
c. Vitamin C deficiency causes scurvy
d. In excess amounts they can be toxic
e. Large supplies can be stored in the liver

15. Thiamine deficiency causes

a. Infantile beri-beri
b. Pyruvate accumulation in the blood
c. Alcoholism
d. Wernicke's encephalopathy
e. Korsakoff's psychosis

16. Pellagra is characterized by

a. Dermatitis
b. Deafness
c. Dyskinesia
d. Diarrhoea
e. Dementia

TCA, tricarboxylic acid; GI, gastrointestinal; NAD, nicotinamide adenine dinucleotide; NADP, nicotinamide adenine dinucleotide phosphate; FAD, flavine adenine dinucleotide; FMN, flavine mononucleotide; CNS, central nervous system

EXPLANATION: WATER-SOLUBLE VITAMINS

A vitamin is a **complex organic substance** required in the diet in **small amounts**, whose absence leads to a **deficiency disease**. Nine vitamins are **water soluble** (**B group** and **C**). They are normally stored in very small amounts and therefore are needed on a regular basis. They are generally not toxic in excess. The B group of vitamins acts as cofactors in the pathways of intermediary metabolism.

Thiamine (B1) is a **coenzyme** in the reaction to convert **pyruvate** to **acetyl CoA**, which enters the TCA cycle. Diet-related thiamine deficiency causes **beri-beri**, which may manifest as infantile, acute cardiac or chronic dry. **Alcohol**-related thiamine deficiency causes **Wernicke-Korsakoff** syndrome, which is the third most common cause of dementia in the US. **Alcohol** consumption causes anorexia and the **inhibition** of **active transport of thiamine across the intestinal wall** as well as the conversion of thiamine to its active form, thiamine pyrophosphate.

NAD and **NADP,** which are important in redox reactions, are derivatives of niacin. Niacin is found in cereals in very small amounts, and is especially poor in maize. **Pellagra** is caused by **niacin** (B group) deficiency. It affects the skin, GI tract and the CNS. Remember the three Ds: dermatitis, diarrhoea and dementia! Pellagra can be cured by increasing the protein content of the diet, because nicotinic acid (niacin) can be formed in the body from tryptophan. Untreated deficiency causes death.

Vitamin	Source	Function	Deficiency disorder
B1 (thiamine)	Wholegrain, pork, poultry	Coenzyme for pyruvate dehydrogenase and 2-oxoglutarate dehydrogenase	Beri-beri Wernicke–Korsakoff syndrome
B2 (riboflavin)	Milk	FAD and FMN in redox reactions	Cheilosis Angular somatitis Glossitis Seborrhoeic dermatitis
Niacin	Cereals	NAD and NADP in redox reactions	Pellagra
B6	Meat, wholegrain	Coenzyme in transamination and decarboxylation of amino acids and glycogen phosphorylase	Convulsions
B12	Animal tissues	1-C transfer reactions	Pernicious anaemia
Folate	Green vegetables, liver		
C (ascorbic acid)	Citrus fruits	Antioxidant Coenzyme in hydroxylation of proline and lysine in collagen formation	Scurvy

Answers

14. F T T F F
15. T T F T T
16. T F F T T

17. Vitamin A

a. Is found in fish liver oils
b. Is crucial to vision in dim light
c. Is transported in chylomicrons from the gut to the liver
d. May cause teratogenicity if taken in excess
e. Controls protein synthesis in cell differentiation

18. True or false? Vitamin E

a. Is a tocopherol
b. Prevents oxidation of polyunsaturated fatty acids
c. Deficiency is common in humans
d. Protects normal prostaglandin metabolism
e. Is in rich supply in human milk

19. Vitamin D

a. Is important for the regulation of Zn^{2+} levels in the blood
b. May be formed from the action of UV light on the skin
c. Is converted in the body to the active form 1,25-dihydroxycholecalciferol
d. If deficient in children's diet will lead to colour blindness
e. May be found in green leaves and fresh vegetables

20. Vitamin K

a. Can be formed by microorganisms in the human gut
b. Is found in cereals and nuts
c. Plays a role in the blood clotting process
d. Is the vitamin most likely to be deficient in new born babies
e. Acts as a cofactor for the carboxylation of glutamate residues in proteins

FA, fatty acid; UV, ultraviolet

EXPLANATION: FAT-SOLUBLE VITAMINS

The **fat-soluble vitamins** are **A, D, E** and **K**. They are usually stored in the body and are not excreted easily if taken in excess.

Vitamin	Source	Function	Deficiency disorder
A (retinol, beta-carotene)	Animal liver, fish liver oils, green, yellow and orange vegetables and fruit	Visual pigments in the retina. Beta-carotene is an antioxidant	Night blindness, xerophthalmia
D (calciferol)	UV light action on 7-dehydrocholesterol in skin	Maintains Ca^{2+} balance in blood	Rickets (children), osteomalacia (adults)
E (tocopherols)	Vegetable oils	Antioxidant in cell membranes	Extremely rare. Infants – haemolytic anaemia
K	Green leafy vegetables and microorganisms in the intestine	Coenzyme in formation of carboxyglutamate in enzymes for blood clotting	Impaired clotting, haemorrhagic disease

Dietary sources of **vitamin A** include **retinol** in **animal liver and fish liver oils, whole milk, egg yolk** and **beta-carotene** in green, yellow and orange vegetables and fruit. The active forms are retinoic acid and retinal. They have an important role in the control of protein synthesis in cell growth and differentiation, as they bind chromatin in the nucleus. **11,*cis*-Retinal** is important in converting light energy to impulses in the optic nerve, and is particularly critical to vision in low light intensity.

Vitamin A is transported from the gut to the liver in **chylomicrons**, and from the liver to the tissues bound to a specific retinal-binding protein or pre-albumin. Deficiency of vitamin A is usually associated with poor protein diets. It is not necessarily reversible by administration of vitamin A alone since the synthesis of retinol-binding protein is affected by the deficiency and therefore so is vitamin A absorption. Deficiency may cause **night blindness, xerophthalmia** and **keratomalacia**. Vitamin A toxicity is unlikely with a normal diet but can cause dermatitis, hair loss, and hepatic dysfunction. In pregnancy it can cause **teratogenicity** if taken in excess.

Vitamin E belongs to a family of compounds called **tocopherols**, which are naturally occurring **antioxidants**. Disruption of polyunsaturated FAs by oxidation disturbs cell membrane structure, integrity and prostaglandin metabolism. **Free radicals** attack polyunsaturated fatty acids to form a peroxyl radical. The peroxyl radical may attack other polyunsaturated FAs, causing a chain reaction. Vitamin E can prevent this happening by reacting with the peroxyl radical to produce FA hydroperoxide. **Although vitamin E becomes a radical itself, it is stable and can be reduced to its original active antioxidant form by vitamin C.** Deficiency is unheard of, apart from in premature low weight babies, as vitamin E is present in most cereals and plant foods.

Answers
17. T T T T T
18. T T F T F
19. F T T F F
20. T F T T F

21. True or false? Iron deficiency anaemia

a. Cannot be reversed by dietary supplementation with Fe^{2+}
b. Is most common in premenopausal women
c. Is often due to a defective Fe^{2+} carrier, transferrin
d. Causes an increase in transferrin levels in plasma
e. May affect the absorption of other trace elements

22. Using a labelled diagram, describe the process of iron uptake in cells

23. Idiopathic haemochromatosis

a. Affects 1 in 20 newborns
b. Causes a ratio of haemosiderin Fe:ferritin Fe of less than 1.0
c. Causes liver failure
d. Is treated with blood transfusions
e. Is caused by increased uptake of Fe^{2+} from the diet

24. Regarding iron

a. The total amount in the body is 30 mg
b. Vitamin C increases its absorption
c. Tea inhibits its absorption
d. Fe^{3+} is taken up by simple endocytosis from the gut lumen
e. Haemochromatosis is more common in men than in women

GI, gastrointestinal; NSAID, non-steroidal anti-inflammatory drug

EXPLANATION: IRON

The tissue richest in iron is blood. **Haemoglobin contains 67 per cent** of the **total body iron** (about 4 g in a healthy adult male). Out of the 10–30 mg that we take in each day, only 10 per cent is absorbed and required. Iron is more readily **absorbed** from the **ferrous (Fe^{2+})** state but most dietary iron is in the ferric (Fe^{3+}) state, so vitamin C in the diet aids in the absorption of iron from foods. Most iron is absorbed in the **upper** part of the **small intestine**. The mucosal cells contain an intracellular carrier. The iron that has been absorbed is then either stored with **ferritin (as Fe^{3+})** or it binds to **transferrin** in the Fe^{2+} state. Transferrin is an iron-transporting polypeptide in the plasma. It carries iron to sites of utilization or storage.

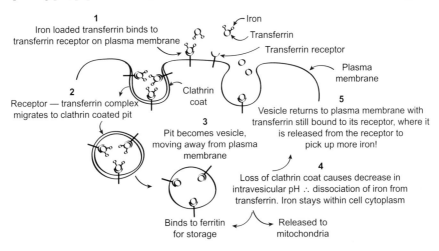

1
Iron loaded transferrin binds to transferrin receptor on plasma membrane

Iron
Transferrin
Transferrin receptor
Plasma membrane

2
Receptor — transferrin complex migrates to clathrin coated pit

Clathrin coat

5
Vesicle returns to plasma membrane with transferrin still bound to its receptor, where it is released from the receptor to pick up more iron!

3
Pit becomes vesicle, moving away from plasma membrane

4
Loss of clathrin coat causes decrease in intravesicular pH ∴ dissociation of iron from transferrin. Iron stays within cell cytoplasm

Binds to ferritin for storage
Released to mitochondria

Iron homeostasis depends on **absorption alone** since there is no physiological mechanism for the secretion of iron in the human body. With increasing iron intake, **ferritin** concentration in mucosal cells **increases** and **transferrin** in the plasma **decreases** so that the transporter becomes saturated and iron is diverted to **storage**. Iron deficiency is the commonest micronutrient deficiency in the world. Since iron is essential for haemoglobin production, a deficiency causes a **reduction** in the rate of **haemoglobin synthesis** and can accordingly result in **anaemia**.

One in 20 people carry the gene for **idiopathic (primary) haemochromatosis**. It is more common in men, since women are protected by menstruation and childbirth. In this disorder an extra 3–4 mg of iron are absorbed per day. As it cannot be excreted, iron accumulates in the liver, pancreas and heart, causing severe liver damage. Ferritin molecules aggregate in deposits in lysosomal membranes, called haemosiderin. Haemosiderin Fe: ferritin Fe ratio increases to 10:1. Treatment involves the removal of 500 mL of blood every week for 1–3 years.

People at risk for iron deficiency include: children/adolescents during phases of rapid growth, anyone with a history of recurrent bleeding, women with heavy periods, people taking aspirin or NSAIDs regularly and patients with GI disease.

Answers

21. F T F T F
22. See diagram
23. F F T F T
24. F T T F T

25. True or false? Calcium

a. Is of major importance to health in growing children
b. Is vital for nerve impulse transmission
c. Plasma levels are raised by calcitonin
d. Plasma levels rise in response to parathyroid hormone
e. Absorption is increased by fibre in the diet

26. Look at the flow diagram below and answer the following questions about vitamin D and calcium homeostasis

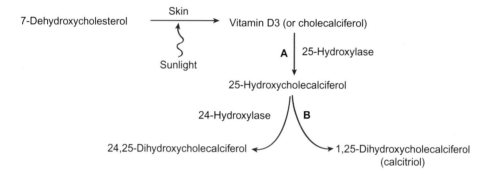

a. Where does reaction **A** take place?
b. Where does reaction **B** take place?
c. Name the missing enzyme that catalyses **B**
d. What effect does the active form of vitamin D have?

27. True or false? Zinc

a. Is found in all tissues in the body
b. Intake should be at least 200 mg/day
c. Deficiency causes hypogonadism
d. Is required for efficient wound healing
e. Is present in high levels in wholemeal bread

EXPLANATION: CALCIUM AND ZINC

Ca^{2+} and PO_4^- are the most **plentiful minerals** in the body. Ninety-nine per cent of the body's Ca^{2+} is found in **bone**, and it is also necessary in the regulation of nerve impulse transmission, muscle contraction, ion transport and blood clotting. Ca^{2+} dietary **requirements** are especially **high** in times **of rapid growth, during infancy, adolescence**, and during **pregnancy** and **lactation**. Ca^{2+} homeostasis is therefore very **tightly regulated** by hormones. The normal range in the plasma is 2.25–2.55 mmol/L. The diet should provide approximately 800 mg Ca^{2+}/day, and higher levels during lactation and pregnancy (120 mg).

Dietary Ca^{2+} is actively absorbed in the mucosal cells of the small intestine. Absorption is dependent on the active metabolite of vitamin D, **calcitriol**. In **vitamin D deficiency** absorption of Ca^{2+} and PO_4^- is severely **impaired (26d)**. Vitamin D also **increases** the release of Ca^{2+} and PO_4^- from bone, and the **reabsorption** of these minerals in the kidney.

Not all dietary Ca^{2+} is available for absorption, some can form insoluble Ca^{2+} salts that cannot be absorbed (e.g. phytic acid/phytate). People with a high phytate diet absorb a lower proportion of their dietary Ca^{2+}.

Other hormones are involved in Ca^{2+} homeostasis. **Parathyroid hormone increases absorption** of Ca^{2+} from the gut by increasing synthesis of 1α-hydroxylase, which activates vitamin D. It also increases **reabsorption** from the kidney. Both effects contribute to increase in plasma Ca^{2+} levels. **Calcitonin** released from the **thyroid gland decreases resorption** of Ca^{2+} from the bone and **inhibits** its **reabsorption** by the kidney and thus lowers plasma levels of Ca^{2+}.

Zinc is the **prosthetic** group for many **enzymes**. It is also incorporated into the receptor proteins for steroid and thyroid hormones, calcitriol and vitamin A. Recommended daily intake of zinc is 10 mg/day. Zinc is found in all tissues of the body, but it is particularly high in the bone, liver and kidney. Zinc deficiency causes growth retardation, decreased wound healing and hypogonadism (i.e. much delayed puberty). It is only normally seen in populations whose diet is based on unleavened wholemeal bread, because wheat flour does not provide much zinc, and that which is available is bound to phytate. Phytate also inhibits the absorption of iron. Zinc depletion may also be caused by drugs such as thiazide and loop diuretics, and alcohol. Zinc deficiency can be successfully treated with replacement zinc therapy.

Answers
25. T T F T F
26. a. Liver; b. Kidney; c. 1α-hydroxylase; d. See explanation
27. T F T T F

SECTION

5 CLINICAL ASPECTS OF NUTRITION

- OBESITY AND NUTRITIONAL HEALTH RISKS   98

- WATER-SOLUBLE VITAMINS – DEFICIENCY
  DISORDERS   100

- EATING DISORDERS   102

- DIET AND DISEASE   104

- ENTERAL AND PARENTERAL NUTRITION,
  AND BREASTFEEDING   106

- HEALTHY EATING   108

- FOOD SENSITIVITIES   110

5 CLINICAL ASPECTS OF NUTRITION

1. The following are considered risk factors for obesity in the UK

a. Low level of education and income
b. Genetic predisposition
c. High birthweight in infancy
d. Low basal metabolic rate
e. Minimal physical activity

2. The following clinical conditions are associated with obesity

a. Cardiovascular disease
b. Asthma
c. Diabetes type II
d. Gallbladder stones
e. Osteoporosis

3. The Barker hypothesis

a. Suggests nutrient availability to a fetus can affect its health in adult life
b. Implies that a high birth weight is bad for your health
c. Is poorly supported by population studies
d. Explains the higher incidence of diabetes mellitus in immigrant populations
e. Is also known as programming

BMI, body mass index; CHD, coronary heart disease

EXPLANATION: OBESITY AND NUTRITIONAL HEALTH RISKS

Obesity can be defined as an **excess store of fat** resulting from the cumulative ingestion of **greater quantities of energy than the body uses**. In order for a man to be obese more than 20 per cent of his body weight must be due to fat. In terms of body mass index (weight/height^2) a BMI between 25 and 30 kg/m^2 indicates overweight, and one of between **30 and 40** kg/m^2 indicates **obesity**. Obesity is more prevalent in **lower socio-economic** classes in western countries, and amongst the affluent classes in the poorer areas of the world. There may also be genetic predisposition in some family pedigrees.

Why is obesity increasing? Because of a combination of **overeating and under-exercising**. Cheaper food, greater advertising, high levels of stress, television and more labour-saving machines are all contributing factors to energy intake being greater than expenditure.

Although obesity is associated with excessive intake compared with nutrient requirement, **basal metabolic rate** is often **higher** in obese people.

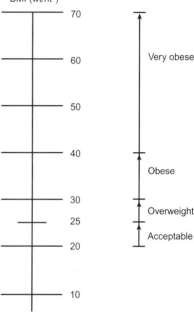

The incidence of CHD correlates with obesity. Between 1 and 5 per cent of health care costs in the UK are attributable to obesity or overweight. If everyone was at their optimum weight there would be 25 per cent fewer CHD cases in the UK. Other conditions associated with obesity are **diabetes type II, cancer, osteoarthritis, gallstones and hypertension**.

The **Barker hypothesis** states that **fetal environment**, particularly maternal nutrition, can alter the physiology of the fetus such that it develops diseases in later life. This is also known as **programming**. **Low birth weight** is associated with **a greater risk of CHD** and **diabetes mellitus**. Individuals are particularly at risk if moving from an area of poor nutrition (experienced in the womb) to good nutrition (experienced as an adult). This is called catch-up growth.

Answers
1. T T F F T
2. T F T T F
3. T F F T T

4. True or false? Folic acid

a. Is found in green leafy vegetables   b. Is important for one-carbon metabolism
c. Deficiency causes haemolytic anaemia   d. Requires vitamin B6 for absorption
e. Intake must be increased during pregnancy

5. Vitamins and blood disorders

a. Explain why vitamin B12 deficiency and folate deficiency produce the same symptoms?
b. Why is it important to take folic acid during pregnancy?

6. True or false? Vitamin C

a. May prevent the common cold   b. Is better absorbed in smokers
c. Inactivates free radicals   d. In megadoses may cause kidney stones
e. Is necessary for collagen synthesis

7. Match the dietary deficiency of the vitamins listed below to the correct disease

Options

A. Haemorrhagic disease of the newborn
B. Wernicke's encephalopathy
C. Pernicious anaemia
D. Angular stomatitis
E. Night blindness
F. Rickets

1. Vitamin D
2. Vitamin K
3. Riboflavin
4. Vitamin B12
5. Thiamine
6. Vitamin A

THF, tetrahydrofolate; NADP, nicotinamide adenine dinucleotide phosphate; NADPH, reduced nicotinamide adenine dinucleotide phosphate; DNA, deoxyribonucleic acid; RBC, red blood cell; NADP+, oxidized form of nicotinamide adenine dinucleotide phosphate

EXPLANATION: WATER-SOLUBLE VITAMINS – DEFICIENCY DISORDERS

Folic acid (folate) is found in green leafy vegetables and is involved in one-carbon metabolism. **Folate supplements** are vital during **pregnancy**. Groups of women who are prescribed folic acid show a significant decrease in the incidence of **neural tube defects** in their newborns **(5b)**.

Megaloblastic anaemia can be caused by a deficiency of **vitamin B12** or a deficiency of **folate**. Symptoms are lethargy, weakness, dizziness, anorexia and neurological changes.

Vitamin B12 is a carrier of **methyl groups** in the conversion of amino acid **homocysteine** to **methionine**. Folate in its active form, THF, is a carrier of 1-carbon fragments, is used to convert homocysteine to methionine or is used in purine and pyrimidine synthesis, for example the formation of thymidylate.
When THF carries a methyl group it can only be converted back to active tetrafolate by passing the methyl group on to vitamin B12. If vitamin B12 is lacking, then THF cannot be recycled, and it is trapped in the methyl form. The consequences of this are that methionine cannot be formed from homocysteine and that methyl THF cannot be used to synthesize thymidylate. Thymidylate is required to carry out DNA elongation. DNA synthesis is therefore inadequate and megaloblastic anaemia (giant RBCs) results **(5a)**.

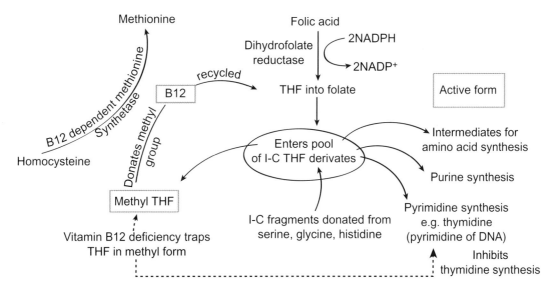

Vitamin C or **ascorbic acid** is a well known **antioxidant** nutrient that functions as a **coenzyme** in hydroxylation reactions for **collagen formation**. It is found in citrus fruits, tomatoes and berries. Severe deficiency leads to scurvy. Intake of approximately 1 g/day decreases the severity of symptoms of colds but does not reduce their incidence. Intakes of over 2 g/day may cause kidney stones due to accumulation of oxalic acid, the end product of vitamin C metabolism.

Answers
4. T T F F T
5. See explanation
6. F F T T F
7. 1 – F, 2 – A, 3 – D, 4 – C, 5 – B, 6 – E (see explanations on pages 89 and 91)

8. The following are features of anorexia nervosa. True or false?

a. Amenorrhea
b. Loss of sex drive
c. Fear of fatness
d. Loss of appetite
e. Purging

9. Anorexia nervosa

a. Affects only women
b. Affects mostly lower social classes
c. Is defined by a BMI of 20–22
d. Can be caused by depression
e. Is more prevalent in white populations

10. Bulimia nervosa is characterized by

a. Rapid weight loss
b. Binge eating
c. Purging
d. Calorie counting
e. Body dissatisfaction

BMI, body mass index

EXPLANATION: EATING DISORDERS

Anorexia nervosa affects **1 per cent** of women, in a ratio of 16 female cases to every male case. It is more prevalent in **white females** in western countries of **higher social classes**. Other features of anorexia include **amenorrhea, loss of libido, body image disturbance, calorie counting and preoccupation with food. 50 per cent of girls with anorexia also vomit or purge**. Hunger is usually present but suppressed.

Girls with anorexia are often high achievers, well-behaved and conformist before they become ill. It is thought that pressure to be perfect, feelings of self-inefficacy and self-doubt may be associated with the disease.

Early diagnosis is vital because long illness and severe weight loss are bad prognostic factors.

Criteria for a diagnosis of anorexia nervosa are:

- BMI under 17.5
- Disturbance of body image
- Refusal to maintain normal weight
- Intense fear of becoming fat
- No known medical illness leading to weight loss.

Bulimia nervosa (or just bulimia) is characterized by a cycle of **bingeing** and **purging**. Binge eating usually occurs when the patient is alone and is characterized by the sense of being out of control and unable to stop eating. Vomiting is an ineffective way to lose calories therefore bulimics are usually of normal weight. The long-term health problems are that the stomach may dilate, and vomiting can cause electrolyte imbalances. Bulimia affects 2–3 per cent of women in the West. The short-term prognosis is generally good.

Both anorexia and bulimia require specialist treatment. Many are treated in the **community** but **hospital admission** may be required, particularly in those who are severely underweight. Patients undergo **psychotherapy** to normalize their eating patterns and to change their perception of their own bodies.

Answers

8. T T T F T
9. F F F T T
10. F T T F T

11. The death rate from cancer could be reduced if more people

a. Stopped smoking
b. Reduced their salt intake
c. Avoided high consumption of saturated fats
d. Avoided drinking and driving
e. Consumed more fresh vegetables and dietary fibre

12. Hypertension is exacerbated by

a. Obesity
b. High alcohol consumption
c. Lack of vitamin C
d. High dietary iodine
e. High dietary Na^+

13. Regular alcohol consumption in excess

a. Correlates with higher plasma concentration of high density lipoprotein
b. Can cause B vitamin deficiencies
c. Is associated with Wernicke–Korsakoff syndrome
d. Can precipitate hypoglycaemia
e. Increases folate absorption

14. Kwashiorkor

a. Is a manifestation of protein-energy malnutrition
b. Is characterized by oedema
c. May occur in combination with marasmus
d. Is most common in South-East Asia
e. Is associated with death by pneumonia

15. Dietary protein requirements

a. The recommended protein requirement for a healthy adult is 0.8g/kg/day
b. An additional 15% protein intake above the recommended intake is needed during pregnancy and lactation
c. Children require at least 8% of their diet from high quality protein sources
d. Men require a higher protein intake than women on a kg body weight basis
e. A low protein intake is recommended during convalescence after major surgery

CHD, coronary heart disease; FA, fatty acid; GI, gastrointestinal; PEM, protein energy malnutrition

EXPLANATION: DIET AND DISEASE

CHD and **cancer** could be **reduced** if more people stopped **smoking, reduced saturated fat intake, consumed five fresh portions of fruit/vegetables a day, followed drinking guidelines** and undertook **regular physical activity**. CHD could also be reduced by reducing Na^+ intake.

Causal factors of essential hypertension include: obesity, anxiety/stress, Na^+ intake and alcohol. **Hypertension** is linked to **obesity** because obese people are thought to have a **higher intake of Na^+**. **Na^+ retention** causes an **increase** in **arteriole smooth muscle tone**. The effect of alcohol intake on blood pressure starts at above three drinks per day. The mechanism has not been established, it is thought to act by increasing red cell volume and therefore blood viscosity. The following dietary components may reduce blood pressure: K^+, Ca^{2+}, polyunsaturated FAs, Mg^{2+} and vegetarianism.

Alcohol has empty calories – it does not provide adequate vitamins and nutrients. For this reason **B vitamin deficiencies** in **alcoholics** can cause **Wernicke–Korsakoff syndrome**. Alcoholics also have **decreased folate** absorption in the small intestine. Binge drinking may cause hypoglycaemia as alcohol intake inhibits gluconeogenesis.

Five million children worldwide die every year from malnutrition. In the UK it is usually precipitated by severe illness, but in developing countries it is more likely to be caused by poor diet. **Kwashiorkor** is most common in rural Africa and is due to deficiency of both protein and foods providing calories (PEM). It is characterized by **painless pitting oedema, skin lesions, muscle wasting and GI infections**. The excess fluid retention (oedema) can often mask loss of body tissue.

The most common cause of death from PEM is **pneumonia**, since these children have defective immune systems and are therefore at increased risk for infection.

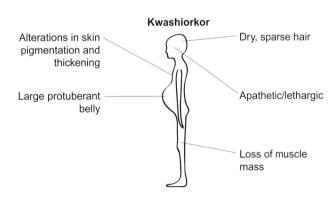

Kwashiorkor

Alterations in skin pigmentation and thickening

Large protuberant belly

Dry, sparse hair

Apathetic/lethargic

Loss of muscle mass

Marasmus is characterized by the loss of lean tissue and **subcutaneous fat**, causing characteristic **wrinkling** of the **skin**. It can be difficult to differentiate from dehydration. It is possible to present with a combination of the two, called marasmic kwashiorkor.

Answers
11. T F T F T
12. T T F F T
13. T T T T F
14. T T T F T
15. T T T F F

16. Regarding enteral nutrition

a. It is cheaper than parenteral nutrition
b. It should be used if the GI tract is functioning normally
c. It requires a centrally placed feeding catheter
d. It carries a high risk of introducing infection
e. It provides all the normal nutrients required in the diet

17. Breastfeeding

a. List and explain two advantages of breastfeeding for infants
b. List and explain two disadvantages of breastfeeding for infants
c. What is meant by 'failure to thrive'?

GI, gastrointestinal; HIV, human immunodeficiency virus; FA, fatty acid; IgA, immunoglobulin A

EXPLANATION: ENTERAL AND PARENTERAL NUTRITION, AND BREASTFEEDING

Patients who are unable to eat or suffer intestinal failure require nutritional support. The table below compares **enteral** and **parenteral nutrition**.

	Enteral	Parenteral
What is it?	Nutrition delivered by tube	Nutrition delivered intravenously
Indications	Anorexia, swallowing disorders, gastric statis, intestinal malfunction	Inflammatory bowel disease, mucositis following chemotherapy, pancreatitis, multi-organ failure
Type of nutrition	Polymeric whole protein foods most common	Solution containing glucose, lipid, amino acids, electrolytes, minerals, vitamins, trace elements
Method	Nasogastric, nasojejunal, percutaneous gastrostomy, percutaneous jejunostomy	Fine bore peripheral cannulae or (for prolonged use) central venous access
Complications	Glucose, electrolyte imbalance, refeeding syndrome, GI symptoms, pneumonia due to aspiration	Glucose, electrolyte imbalance, catheter-related infection, liver and bilary disease, enterocyte atrophy

Breast milk is generally regarded as the **best diet** for **babies**, rather than cow's milk, for two main reasons:

• Breast milk has **anti-infective properties**. Secretory IgA comprises 90 per cent of breast milk immunoglobulin. It also contains lysozyme (a bacteriolytic enzyme), lactoferrin (inhibits the growth of *Escherichia coli*) and interferon (an antiviral agent). Breast milk also contains phagocytic macrophages and lymphocytes. GI infection is known to be less common in breastfed babies
• Breast milk has good **nutritional properties**. It has a high protein quality, is hypoallergenic and is very rich in oleic acid, a monounsaturated FA. Long chain FAs aid neurological development. Other advantages are that it promotes **emotional attachment** between **mother** and **baby**, and it can **reduce** the **risk** of **breast cancer (17a)**.

The occasonal disadvantages of breast milk are less well known. It is possible to transmit **infection** (e.g. HIV) as well as drugs through breast milk. Breastfeeding can cause a mild self-limiting hyperbilirubinaemia, resulting in jaundice. It can also be associated with a **vitamin K deficiency** as there are insufficient levels in breast milk **(17b)**.

Failure to thrive is the term used to describe babies who demonstrate suboptimal weight gain/growth **(17c)**. Causes are traditionally divided into organic and non-organic. Non-organic causes are associated with psychosocial and environmental factors. Organic causes include inadequate food intake, chronic illness and diminished absorption of consumed food.

Answers
16. T T F F T
17. See explanation

18. Special dietary requirements

    a. Name two nutritional deficiencies that may occur on a vegan diet
    b. Suggest three dietary guidelines of particular benefit to the elderly

19. Case study

A slightly overweight 44-year-old city worker comes to see his GP because he is concerned about his heart. He has recently been experiencing exertional chest pain. After talking with him, it transpires that his father died from a heart attack at the age of 50. What kind of **dietary** advice would you give this man?

20. Case study

An elderly Asian woman comes to see her GP complaining of bone pain and general fatigue. On examination he notes that there is weakness and wasting in her proximal limb muscles. Her blood test reveals low plasma Ca^{2+}, and a raised alkaline phosphatase.

    a. What is likely to be the cause of this patient's symptoms?
    b. How would the diagnosis be confirmed?
    c. What might be a consequence of her low plasma Ca^{2+}?
    d. What would an X-ray of the woman's bones show?

CHD, coronary heart disease; LDL, low density lipoprotein; FA, fatty acid; GP, general practitioner; UV, ultraviolet

EXPLANATION: HEALTHY EATING

There is a general perception in western society that vegetarians are healthier than meat-eaters. However, it really depends on the degree of vegetarianism being adhered to. **Vegans** who eat no animal products (including eggs and dairy) are at risk of **vitamin B12 deficiency**. Supplements are therefore essential for vegans who are pregnant and for infants. Vegans also may be **Ca^{2+} deficient** since they lack good sources such as milk, yoghurt and cheese **(18a)**.

The only nutritional risk to **vegetarians** who eat milk and eggs is **iron deficiency**. Generally it is believed that vegetarians have a lower risk of obesity, CHD and hypertension.

Elderly people are at risk of **nutritional deficiency** in the western world, probably more due to social and environmental factors than anything else. Sensible advice to avoid nutritional deficiency includes the following:

- Women should maintain a high intake of Ca^{2+} from **dairy products** to help delay osteoporosis
- People who are **housebound** or **immobile** should take daily prophylactic supplements of **vitamin D**
- Eating **fatty fish** or taking **fish oil supplements** can prevent **thrombosis**
- Eating plenty of fruit and vegetables will maintain a **high fibre content** in the diet. This prevents constipation, which is often a problem for elderly people **(18b)**.

The three main risk factors for **CHD** are: smoking, hypertension and high plasma LDL-cholesterol plasma.

CHD can be prevented to some extent by controlling risk factors. **Hypertension** and **plasma cholesterol** are both affected by the diet. Advice to patients with a family history of coronary heart disease would include suggesting a **cholesterol check**, and, depending on the results, **reducing saturated fat intake** to around 8–10 per cent of the diet. **Omega-3 polyunsaturated FAs** (found in seafoods and rapeseed oils) should be increased in the diet since they lower LDL-cholesterol. **Monounsaturated fats** (in olive oil) should also be **increased**, but total fat should not exceed 30 per cent of the dietary intake. **Hypertension** can be reduced by **restricting salt intake (19)**.

Bone and joint pain in the elderly are characteristic of **osteomalacia**, probably due to **vitamin D deficiency** caused by poor exposure to **sunlight** together with **a dietary deficiency of Ca^{2+} (20a)**. Osteomalacia and rickets are more common in Asian immigrants in the UK than in other ethnic populations. This is thought to be because chapati flour contains phytate, which binds Ca^{2+}. Deeply pigmented skins generate less vitamin D in response to UV light exposure than paler skins. The diagnosis can be confirmed by measuring 25-hydroxy vitamin D in the plasma **(20b)**. The patient's low plasma Ca^{2+} may cause a secondary hyperparathyroidism – raised parathyroid hormone **(20c)**. Radiological studies would show bones appearing less dense than normal, with localized areas of decalcification on the concave surface (pseudofractures) **(20d)**.

Answers

18. See explanation
19. See explanation
20. See explanation

21. Food hypersensitivity

a. Describe how food sensitivity can be diagnosed
b. List three different food types that may cause anaphylaxis as an allergic reaction
c. List three food types that may trigger migraine

22. Case study

A 34-year-old man presents to his GP complaining of chronic diarrhoea. For the past year he has been passing two–three stools a day that are pale, smell awful and are difficult to flush away. He has lost 2 stone in weight over the past year as well. On examination the man has a papular itchy rash on his back and several mouth ulcers. A blood test reveals low folate and vitamin B12.

a. Why are his stools pale and difficult to flush?
b. Why is he anaemic?
c. How can this man be treated?

23. Concerning lactose intolerance

a. Lactose is digested in the healthy small intestine to one molecule of glucose and one molecule of galactose
b. Babies with a genetic deficiency of lactase will thrive on human breast milk, but not on cow's milk
c. Biofermented yoghurt contains a higher lactose content than fresh milk
d. True lactase deficiency can be confirmed by the 'hydrogen breath test'
c. Temporary secondary lactose intolerance may occur after a severe gastrointestinal infection

GI, gastrointestinal; GP, general practitioner; IgE, immunoglobulin E

EXPLANATION: FOOD SENSITIVITIES

There are no clear-cut diagnostic tests for food sensitivity. **Skin tests** are a common and simple method. Drops of the extract of the **allergen** are administered to the **skin** through a pinprick. A positive response is recorded if the skin **wheals and flares within 20 minutes**. This is an indication that IgE specific to the food allergen sits on the surface of the mast cells **(21a)**. See also page 112 for a further explanation.

Dietary manipulation may give diagnostic information about all types of food sensitivity. For example, a patient may keep a **diet diary** together with a **symptom diary**, although this is subject to bias. An **elimination diet** involves the elimination for two or three weeks of all foods that are thought to provoke sensitivity. Foods are then reintroduced slowly one by one to identify the allergen. Elimination diets do carry the risk of nutritional deficiency **(21a)**.

Foods that can cause anaphylaxis include **peanuts, cow's milk, shellfish, wheat, legumes** and **citrus fruits (21b)**. Reactions occur very quickly: the lips, tongue and mouth **swell up** and itch within minutes, followed by **oedema** of the larynx and bronchi, causing difficulty in breathing, and an acute drop in blood pressure, which can be **very dangerous**. Treatment is with adrenaline.

Migraines are commonly associated with stress, but have many precipitants including **food**. Common triggers are chocolate, cheese, citrus fruits, red wine and sausages **(21c)**.

Patients with coeliac disease show the symptoms associated with **malabsorption**, often characterized by **steatorrhoea** (pale stools that float because of their high fat content) **(22a)**. Malabsorption may have any number of causes, one of which is **coeliac disease**, a **gluten-sensitive** enteropathy. This disorder results in loss of villi, crypt hyperplasia and **chronic inflammation** of the **small bowel mucosa**. The immature cells of the small intestine are unable to absorb nutrients or to produce GI hormones. This reduces **pancreatic** and **bile secretion**, which **impedes fat absorption** in the gut. Anaemia is caused by the folate and B12 deficiency due to impaired absorption **(22b)**. Treatment of coeliac disease is by a **gluten-free diet**, **steroids** (to treat inflammation) and **immunosuppressants (22c)**. People with unrecognized and untreated coeliac disease may have an increased risk of small bowel carcinoma.

Lactose is a disaccharide (composed of glucose and galactose) present in **human and animal milk**, and is an important source of calories for the newborn. It is digested by the enzyme **lactase present in the brush border** of epithelial cells lining the small intestine. Genetic absence of lacatase (from birth) is rare, but most adults of Asian or oriental background lose the ability to express the enzyme during childhood. Severe infections of the GI tract can result in temporary loss of the lactase enzyme. Milk products should be avoided, but yoghurt can be a useful source of Ca^{2+}, with lower levels of lactose. Lactose deficiency can be diagnosed by the hydrogen breath test as the undigested lactose is fermented by microorganisms in the intestine to a variety of products, including CO_2 and H_2.

Answers

21. See explanation
22. See explanation
23. T F F T T

EXPLANATION: FOOD SENSITIVITIES (CONT.)

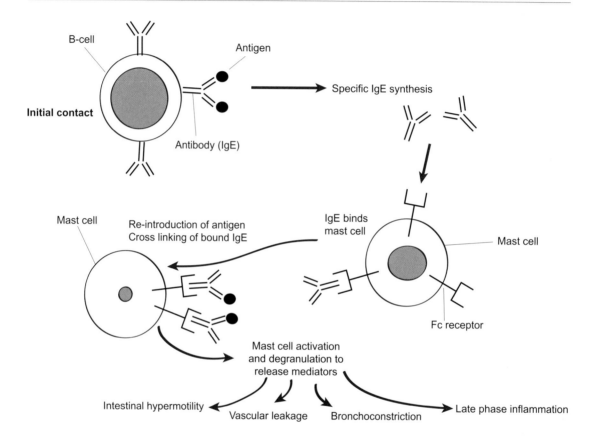

In line with this method, a **radioimmunoassay** may be performed on the serum to show the presence of IgE specific to the food allergen. The problem with these tests is that the presence of IgE antibodies does not necessarily mean that the patient is clinically allergic to the allergen. Conversely, a negative skin test does not exclude food sensitivity mediated by a mechanism other than IgE.

IgE, immunogloblin E

INDEX

amino groups 49, 61
aminotransferases 46, 47, 61
ammonia 48, 49
amphipathic substances 29
amylo-1,6-glucosidase 15
amytal 21
anabolism 71
anaemia 67, 111
   haemolytic 7, 69
   iron deficiency 92, 93
   megaloblastic 101
anaerobic conditions 5, 61, 63
anaphylaxis 111
anorexia 89
anorexia nervosa 102, 103
antioxidants 91, 101
apoA-1 41
apoB100 41
apolipoprotein reservoir 41
apolipoprotein-C2 deficiency 67
apoproteins 41
arachidonic acid 31, 83
arginase 61
arginine 61
arterial smooth muscle 105
arthritis 67, 99
ascorbic acid (vitamin C) 89, 91, 100
aspartate 49, 61, 63
aspartate aminotransferase (AST) 47, 61
atheroma formation 83
atherosclerosis 41, 83
ATP synthase 21
attachment formation 107
autoimmune diseases 67
   endocrine 75, 77

bacteria, intestinal 49
Barker hypothesis 98, 99
basal metabolic rate (BMR) 2, 3, 81, 99
beri-beri 89
beta-carotene 91
bicarbonate 75
biguanides 77
bile 41, 83
bilirubin 69
bingeing 103
biomolecules 58–9
birth weight, low 99
1,6-bisphosphate 9

2,3-bisphosphoglycerate (2,3-BPG) 67
bleeding, recurrent 93
blindness 87
blood
   lipids in 37, 41
   pH 45, 75
   portal 7
blood disorders 100, 101
   see also anaemia
blood-brain barrier 5
body fat 57, 105
   see also obesity
body image disturbance 103
body mass index (BMI) 77, 99
body surface area 3
body temperature 3
bone 95, 109
brain 45, 63, 71, 73, 75
breast cancer 107
breastfeeding 106–7
   see also lactation
buffering capacity 75
bulimia nervosa 102, 103

calcitonin 95
calcitrol 95
calcium
   dietary 94–5, 109
   and glycogen storage 15
calorie counting 103
cancer 99, 104, 105, 107, 111
   see also carcinogens
carbamoyl phosphate 49
carbamoyl phosphate synthetase I 48, 49
carbohydrates 35, 70, 84–5
carbon 85
carbon dioxide 5, 17, 49, 63
carbon monoxide 21
carcinogens 85
carcinoma, small intestine 111
carnitine 31
carnitine shuttle 71
catabolism 56, 57, 71, 75
catecholamines 71, 75
cereals 85, 89
cerebrovascular disease 75
cholesterol 31, 34, 38–9
   checks 109
   dietary influences 83

cholesterol *cont.*
   and lipid transport 41
   synthesis 37
chromatin 91
chylomicrons 40, 41, 71, 91
citrate 11, 19, 35, 59, 61
citrate synthase 19
citric acid cycle (TCA cycle) 5, 16–19
   in diabetics 75
   and the fasting state 71
   and fatty acid metabolism 31
   and the fed state 71
   and gluconeogenesis 25
   intermediates 23, 53
   and ketone bodies 45
   location 59
   metabolic importance 18–19
clathrin 41
CoA 63
coeliac disease 111
coenzymes 49, 89, 101
colds 101
collagen formation 101
coma 5
community care 103
-COOH groups 29
coronary heart disease 99, 105, 109
cortisol 73
covalent modification 15
crystal deposition 67
Cushing's disease 87
cutaneous vasoconstriction 3
cyanide 21
cyclic adenosine monophosphate (cAMP) 15, 23
cytochrome oxidase complex 21
cytosol 59, 63
   and amino acid metabolism 49
   and fatty acid synthesis 35, 37
   and gluconeogenesis 25
   and glucose 6-phosphate 61
   and glucose metabolism 5
   and glycogen synthesis 13
   and glycolysis 9

daily energy expenditure 80, 81
dairy products 109
   see also eggs; milk, cow's
death
   and hypoglycaemia 5

and obesity 99
decarboxylation 16, 17
dehydration 45
dementia 89
dental caries 85
diabetes mellitus 45, 87, 99
   prevalence 75
   symptoms 75, 77
   Type I (insulin dependent) 67, 73, 74–7
   Type II (non-insulin dependent) 67, 74–7
diet 49
   and disease 104–5
   healthy 108–9
diet diaries 111
dietary deficiency 86, 87
dietary manipulation 111
dietary reference values (DRVs) 80, 81
dietary requirements 80, 81
dihydrolipoyl dehydrogenase 17
dihydroxyacetone phosphate 9
2,4-dinitrophenol 21
disaccharides 85, 111
diuresis, osmotic 45
DNA elongation 101
double bonds 29
drugs, breast milk transmission 107

eating disorders 102–3
eggs 91
elderly people 109
electron transport chain 19, 21, 63, 65
electrons 21, 63
elimination diets 111
emotional state 3
endocrinological dysfunction 75, 77, 87
endoplasmic reticulum 39
   rough 41
energy expenditure, daily 80, 81
energy metabolism 2–26
   citric acid cycle 16–19
   gluconeogenesis 22–5
   glucose metabolism 4–5
   glycogen 12–15
   glycolysis 4, 5–11
   metabolic rate 2–3
   oxidative phosphorylation 20–1
enoyl-CoA hydratase 37
enteral nutrition 106–7
enzyme cofactors 62–3

enzyme substrates 60–1
enzymes 3, 5, 23, 31
    of the cholesterol synthesis pathway 39
    disorders 15, 66–9
    reactions 60–1
    and zinc 95
erythrocytes (red blood cells) 65
    enzyme disorders 67, 69
    fuel 7, 71
estimated average requirement (EAR) 80, 81
exocytosis 41

FADH$_2$ (reduced form of flavine adenine dinucleotide) 17,
        19, 21, 33
'failure to thrive' 107
fasting (post-absorptive state) 23, 70–3
fat
    see also lipid metabolism
    body 57, 105
    dietary 82–3, 111
    impeded absorption 111
    oxidation 59
    saturated 29, 30, 83, 105, 109
    subcutaneous 105
fatty acids 25, 28–35, 41, 45
    cells unable to oxidize 30, 31
    cis-unsaturated 83
    essential 28, 30, 31, 82, 83
    in the fasting state 71
    in the fed state 71
    mono-unsaturated 29, 83, 109
    as muscular fuel 75
    oxidation 31, 32–3, 37
    poly-unsaturated 29, 82, 83, 91, 109
    saturated 29, 30, 83
    short-chain 31
    in the starving state 73
    synthesis 34–5, 37, 71
    trans-unsaturated 83
    unsaturated 29, 83
Fe^{2+} 93
Fe^{3+} 93
fed (absorptive) states 3, 7, 70–1
feedback inhibition 39
ferritin 93
fibre, dietary 84, 85, 109
fish 109
fish oils 91, 109
flavine adenine dinucleotide (FAD) 16

folate 101, 105, 111
folic acid 100, 101
food preoccupation 103
food sensitivity 110–12
free radicals 91
fructose 9, 85
fructose 1,6bisphosphatase 23
fruit 85, 91, 105, 109, 111
fuel storage 56, 57

gastrointestinal infections 93, 105, 107, 111
-*genesis* 57
genetic disorders 6, 7, 15
glucagon 15, 23, 39, 71, 75
glucokinase 5, 6, 7
gluconeogenesis 11, 22–5, 61, 71, 73, 75
glucose 25
    blood levels 71, 75
    cellular damage of 5
    conversion of amino acids to 85
    metabolism 4–5, 23, 26
    phosphorylation 7, 59, 61
    qualities 5
    sparing of 71
    in the urine 75
    water solubility 5
α-D glucose 13
glucose-6-phosphatase 23, 67
glucose-6-phosphate 11, 13, 15, 61, 63
glucose-6-phosphate dehydrogenase (G6PD) 65, 67, 68–9
α-glucosidase 77
glucosyl residues 13
GLUT transporters 5
glutamate 47–9, 61
L-glutamate 47
glutamate dehydrogenase 49
glutamine 49
glutathione 65, 69
glutathione peroxidase 65
gluten-free diets 111
gluten-sensitivity 111
glyceraldehyde 3-phosphate 9
glycerol 41, 61, 73, 75
    in the fasting state 71
    in the fed state 71
    and gluconeogenesis 23, 25
    and lipid synthesis 37
    and triglycerides 31
glycerol phosphate 37

glycerol 3-phosphate 9, 25, 61
glycerol 3-phosphate shuttle 63
glycerol kinase 37, 61
glycine 37
glycogen 12–15
    chains 15
    degradation 14, 15, 71
    disorders of storage 14–15, 67
    granules 57
    hepatic stores 23, 57, 73, 77
    muscular stores 57
    structure 12–13
    synthesis 12–13, 15, 59, 71
glycogen phosphorylase 15
glycogen synthase 13, 15
glycogenin 13
glycogenolysis (glycogen degradation) 14, 15, 71
glycolysis 4, 5–11, 37
    in the fed state 71
    intermediates 23, 67
    irreversible reactions 23, 25, 61
    liver reactions 7
    location 59
    regulation 10–11
    reversible reactions 23
α 1,4 glycosidic bonds 13
glycosuria 75
glycotysis 19
Golgi bodies 41
gout 67
growth 81, 93, 95
    catch-up 99
    failure 87
guanosine triphosphate (GTP) 17

haemochromatosis, idiopathic 92, 93
haemoglobin 93
haemolysis 69
haemosiderin 93
healthy eating 108–9
heart disease
    coronary 99, 105, 109
    ischaemic 67, 75
height 3
Heinz bodies 69
hepatocytes 49
hexokinase 5, 7, 11, 59, 61
hexose monophosphate pathway 35
high density lipoprotein (HDL) 41, 42

homocysteine 101
hormone-sensitive lipase 71
hospital admission 103
housebound people 109
hunger 103
hydrogen 85
hydrogen peroxide 65, 67, 69
hydrophilic groups 29, 37
hydrophobic groups 29, 37
3-hydroxy-3-methylglutaryl CoA (HMG CoA) 38, 39
3-hydroxy-3-methylglutaryl CoA reductase 39
3-hydroxybutyrate 73
1-α-hydroxylase 95
hyperammonaemia 49
hyperglycaemia 7, 75, 77
hyperlipidaemias 67
    Goldstein 67
    Type I (Fredrickson) 67
    Type IIa (familial hypercholesterolaemia) 67
hyperparathyroidism 109
hypersensitivity 110
hypertension 99, 104, 105, 109
hyperventilation 75
hypoglycaemia 5, 77
hypoglycaemics, oral 77

immobile people 109
immunoglobulin A (IgA) 107
immunoglobulin E (IgE) 111, 112
immunosuppressants 111
infancy 95
infections
    breast milk transmission 107
    gastrointestinal 93, 105, 107, 111
inflammation 111
insulin 39, 67, 71, 73
    deficiency 75, 77, 87
    resistance 67, 75, 77, 87
    therapy 77
insulin:glucagon ratio 71
interferon 107
intermediate density lipoprotein (IDL) 41
intestinal bacteria 49
iron
    absorption 93
    deficiency 93, 109
    dietary 81, 92–3
    ferric state 93
    ferrous state 93

homeostasis 93
   total body 93
ischaemic heart disease 67, 75
islets of Langerhans 75, 77
isocitrate 17, 59
isocitrate dehydrogenase 19
isoleucine 37
isomerism 59

jaundice 69, 107

keratomalacia 91
α-keto acid 23, 47, 61
ketoacidosis 75, 77, 85
3-ketoacyl-CoA transferase 57, 73
α-ketoglutarate 17, 61
α-ketoglutarate dehydrogenase 19
ketonaemia 44, 45
ketone bodies
   synthesis (ketogenesis) 44–5, 71, 72, 73, 75, 77
   utilization 44, 73
ketonuria 44, 45, 75
kidney
   calcium reabsorption 95
   fatty acid synthesis 35
   gluconeogenesis 23, 25
   glutamate dehydrogenase 49
   in the starved state 73
   urea cycle 49
   zinc reabsorption 95
K_m, high 7
Kreb's cycle *see* citric acid cycle
Kussmaul breathing 75
kwashiorkor 87, 104, 105

lactase 111
lactate 5, 23, 61, 63, 71
lactate dehydrogenase 61
lactation 35, 81, 95
   see also breastfeeding
lactoferrin 107
lactose 85
lactose intolerance 110, 111
lanosterol 39
LCAT 41
legumes 111
leucine 53
linoleic acid 28, 29, 31, 83
linolenic acid 29, 31, 83

lipase, hormone-sensitive 71
lipid metabolism 28–43
   see also fat; fatty acids
   biologically important lipids 36, 37
   cholesterol 38–9
   lipid transport 40–1
   lipogenesis 36–7
   lipoproteins 40–3
   neutral lipids 41
lipoamide reductasetransacetylase 17
lipolysis 75
lipoprotein lipase 41, 67, 71
lipoproteins 40, 41, 42–3, 67
   high density lipoprotein (HDL) 41, 42
   intermediate density lipoprotein (IDL) 41
   low density lipoprotein (LDL) 40, 41, 83, 109
   very low density lipoprotein (VLDL) 41
liver 7, 15, 31, 63
   amino acid metabolism 49
   animal 91
   fasting 70, 71
   and fatty acids synthesis 35
   and G6PD deficiency 69
   general metabolism 56, 57
   gluconeogenesis 23, 25
   and glutamate dehydrogenase 49
   glycogen stores 23, 57, 73, 77
   and glycolysis 71
   and ketogenesis 45
   and lipid synthesis 37
   and lipid transport 41
   in the starved state 73
   zinc and 95
loop diuretics 95
low density lipoprotein (LDL) 41, 83, 109
   receptors 40, 41
lysine 47, 53
-*lysis* 57
lysozyme 107

macrovascular complications 75
malabsorption 111
malate 17, 25, 35, 61, 63
malate dehydrogenase 25, 61, 63
malate-aspartate shuttle 9, 61, 62, 63
malnutrition 86, 87, 105
malonyl-CoA 35, 37, 71
maltose 85
mammary glands 35

marasmic kwashiorkor 105
marasmus 87, 105
margarine 83
Mediterranean diet 82, 83
menstruation 81, 93
metabolic disorders
    diabetes 45, 67, 73, 74–7, 87, 99
    enzyme disorders 66–9
metabolic pathways 58–9
metabolic rate
    basal 2, 3, 81, 99
    factors affecting 2–3
metabolic reactions 58–9
metabolism, general 56–7
metformin 77
methionine 101
methyl groups 101
mevalonic acid 39
microvascular complications 75
migraines 111
milk
    breast 107
    cow's 91, 109, 111
mitochondria 59, 61, 63
    and amino acid metabolism 49
    and the citric acid cycle 17
    fatty acids in 31, 33, 35, 71
    and gluconeogenesis 25
    and glucose metabolism 5
    and the starved state 73
mitochondrial membrane 35
monoacylglycerol 41
monosaccharides 85
mother-baby bonding 107
multi-enzyme complexes 35
muscle 31
    arterial smooth 105
    cardiac 63
    exertion 3
    fuel 71, 73, 75
    glycogen storage 57
    protein breakdown 73
    skeletal 63
    wasting 105

NAD$^+$ (nicotinamide adenine dinucleotide) 9, 17, 61, 63,
    89
NADH (reduced form of nicotinamide adenine dinu-
    cleotide) 9, 17, 19, 21, 33, 49, 61, 63, 65

NADP (nicotinamide adenine dinucleotide phosphate)
    89
NADPH (reduced form of nicotinamide adenine dinu-
    cleotide phosphate) 35, 39, 49, 64–5, 67, 69
nephropathy 75
neural tube defects 101
neuropathy 75
NH^4 49
niacin 89
night blindness 91
nitrogen
    balance 86, 87
    metabolism 47
    removal 49
non-steroidal anti-inflammatory drugs (NSAIDs) 93
noradrenaline 73
nucleosides 63
nutritional deficiency 109, 111
nutritional measurements 80–1

obesity 98–9, 105, 109
oedema 105, 111
oleic acid 107
omega-3 fatty acids 109
omega-6 fatty acids 29
ornithine 61
osteoarthritis 99
osteomalacia 87, 109
overeating 99
overweight persons 99
    see also obesity
oxaloacetate 19, 23, 25, 35, 60, 61, 63, 71
oxidation 32–3, 45
β-oxidation 31, 32, 33, 37
oxidative deamination 48, 49
oxidative phosphorylation 17, 20–1, 59
oxidative reactions 64–5
oxidative stress 69
oxygen 5, 85
oxygen consumption 3
oxygen desaturation curves 67
oxygen intermediates 69

palmitate 35
pancreatic cells
    alpha 75
    beta 67, 75, 77
parathyroid hormone 95, 109
parenteral nutrition 107

peanuts 111
pellagra 88, 89
pentose phosphate pathway 62, 63, 65, 67, 69
peripheral vascular disease 75
peroxyl radicals 91
pH 21, 45, 75
phenylalanine 53
phenylalanine hydroxylase 53, 67
phenylketonuria 52, 53, 67
phosphoenolpyruvate carboxykinase 25, 61
phosphoenolpyruvate (PEP) 7, 23, 25, 61
phosphofructokinase 5, 11
phospholipids 37, 41
phosphorylation 7, 15, 23, 37, 61
    oxidative 17, 20–1, 59
physical exercise 99, 105
    see also activity
phytates 95, 109
pneumonia 105
polydipsia 75, 77
polymers 13
polysaccharides, non-starch 85
polyuria 75, 77
porphyrins 17
portal blood 7
pregnancy 81, 91, 95, 101
programming 99
prosthetic groups 95
protein
    complementation 87
    dietary 86–7, 104
    and fatty acid synthesis 35
    high-quality 87
    synthesis 91
    turnover 46–7
protein kinase 15
protein kinase A 23
protein-energy malnutrition (PEM) 87
protons 21
psychotherapy 103
purging (vomiting) 103
purines 49, 62, 63, 101
pyrimidine 49, 101
pyruvate 45, 53, 61
    acetyl-CoA synthesis 63, 71, 89
    carboxylation 24, 25
    cytosolic conversion to malate 25
    decarboxylation 16, 17
    and gluconeogenesis 23, 25

    and glucose metabolism 4–5
    and glycolysis 7
pyruvate carboxylase 25
pyruvate decarboxylase 17
pyruvate dehydrogenase 37, 61
pyruvate dehydrogenase complex 16, 17, 62, 63
pyruvate kinase 23, 61
    deficiency 6, 7, 67
    and glucose metabolism 5
    and glycolysis 7, 11

radioimmunoassays 112
rate limiting step 39
reference nutrient intake (RNI) 80, 81
retinal 91
11,*cis*-retinal 91
retinoic acid 91
retinol 91
retinopathy 75
ribulose 5-phosphate 63
rickets 109
rotenone 21

scurvy 101
serine 37
shellfish 111
shivering 3
skin lesions 105
skin test 111, 112
skin wrinkling 1–5
small intestine 93, 111
smoking 105, 109
socio-economic groups
    higher 103
    lower 99
sodium intake 105, 109
special dietary requirements 108
specific dynamic action 3
squalene 39
staple foods 80
starch 85
starvation 45, 70, 72–3
steatorrhoea 111
steroids 37, 95, 111
stools, pale 111
succinyl-CoA 17
sucrose 85
sugars 84, 85
sulfonylureas 77

sunlight 109
symptom diaries 111

TCA cycle *see* citric acid cycle
temperature, environmental/body 3
teratogenicity 91
tetrahydrofolate (THF) 101
thermic effect of food 81
thiamine (vitamin B1) 63
    deficiency 88, 89
thiamine pyrophosphate 63, 89
thiazide 95
thiophorase 45
thirst, intense 75
threonine 47
thrombosis 109
thymidylate 101
thyroid gland 95
thyroid hormones 3, 95
thyroxine 3
tocopherols 91
trace elements 85
transamination 47
transferrin 93
triacylglycerol (TAG) 71
    in diabetics 75
    and fatty acid synthesis 35
    and gluconeogenesis 23
    and lipid synthesis 36, 37
    and lipid transport 41
    in the starved state 73
tricarboxylic acid (TCA) cycle *see* citric acid cycle
triglycerides 25, 31
    dietary 83
    hydrolysis 61
    synthesis 59
tyrosine 53

under-exercising 99
uracil diphosphate (UDP) 13
uracil triphosphate (UTP) 13
urea cycle 48, 49, 50–1, 61
uric acid 63, 67, 73

vasoconstriction 3
vegans 109
vegetables 85, 91, 105, 109
vegetarians 109
very low density lipoprotein (VLDL) 41
vision 91
vitamin A 83, 90, 91, 95
    deficiency 87, 91
    toxicity 91
vitamin B1 (thiamine) 63
    deficiency 88, 89
vitamin B6 47
vitamin B12 101, 109, 111
vitamin B group 89, 105
vitamin C (ascorbic acid) 89, 91
    deficiency 100
vitamin D 83, 90, 91
    and calcium 94, 95
    deficiency 87, 95, 109
    supplementation 109
vitamin E 83, 90, 91
vitamin K 83, 90, 91
    deficiency 107
vitamin deficiency diseases 88, 89, 100–1
vitamins
    definition 89
    fat-soluble 83, 90–1
    water-soluble 88–9, 100–1
vomiting, induced 103
von Gierke's disease 67

water 21
weight 3
    see also birth weight
weight loss 75
Wernicke-Korsakoff syndrome 89, 105
wheat 111

xerophthalmia 91

zinc, dietary 94–5